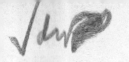

LANGUAGE AWARENESS
FOR TEACHERS

D0912739

Open University Press

English, Language, and Education series

General Editor: Anthony Adams

Lecturer in Education, University of Cambridge

This series is concerned with all aspects of language in education
from the primary school to the tertiary sector. Its authors are
experienced educators who examine both principles and practice of
English subject teaching and language across the curriculum in the
context of current educational and societal developments.

TITLES IN THE SERIES

Narrative and Argument
Richard Andrews (ed.)

Time for Drama
Roma Burgess and Pamela Gaudry

Computers and Literacy
Daniel Chandler and Stephen Marcus (eds)

Readers, Texts, Teachers
Bill Corcoran and Emrys Evans (eds)

Thinking Through English
Paddy Creber

Developing Response to Poetry
Patrick Dias and Michael Hayhoe

Developing English
Peter Dougill (ed.)

The Primary Language Book
Peter Dougill and Richard Knott

Children Talk About Books: Seeing Themselves as Readers
Donald Fry

Literary Theory and English Teaching
Peter Griffith

Lesbian and Gay Issues in the English Classroom
Simon Harris

Reading and Response
Mike Hayhoe and Stephen Parker (eds)

Assessing English
Brian Johnston

Lipservice: The Story of Talk in Schools
Pat Jones

The English Department in a Changing World
Richard Knott

Oracy Matters
Margaret MacLure, Terry Phillips and Andrew Wilkinson (eds)

Language Awareness for Teachers
Bill Mittins

Beginning Writing
John Nicholls et al.

Teaching Literature for Examinations
Robert Protherough

Developing Response to Fiction
Robert Protherough

Microcomputers and the Language Arts
Brent Robinson

English Teaching from A–Z
Wayne Sawyer, Anthony Adams and Ken Watson

Collaboration and Writing
Morag Styles (ed.)

Reconstructing 'A' Level English
Patrick Scott

Reading Within and Beyond the Classroom
Dan Taverner

Reading for Real
Barrie Wade (ed.)

English Teaching in Perspective
Ken Watson

Spoken English Illuminated
Andrew Wilkinson et al.

The Quality of Writing
Andrew Wilkinson

The Writing of Writing
Andrew Wilkinson (ed.)

LANGUAGE AWARENESS FOR TEACHERS

Bill Mittins

Open University Press
Milton Keynes · Philadelphia

Open University Press
Celtic Court
22 Ballmoor
Buckingham MK18 1XW

and
1900 Frost Road, Suite 101
Bristol, PA 19007, USA

First Published 1991

British Library Cataloguing in Publication Data
Mittins, Bill
  Language awareness for teachers. – (English, language and
  education series).
  1. Schools. Curriculum subjects. Language skills. Teaching.
  I. Title   II. Series
  407.1

  ISBN 0-335-09559-3

Library of Congress Cataloging-in-Publication Data

Mittins, William Henry.
  Language awareness for teachers / Bill Mittins.
      p.   cm.—(English, language, and education series)
  Includes bibliographical references and index.
  ISBN 0-335-09559-3
  1. English language—Study and teaching—Great Britain.
  I. Title. II. Series.
  LB1576.M54 1990
  428′.007′041—dc20   90-38823 CIP

Typeset by Rowland Phototypesetting Limited
Bury St Edmunds, Suffolk
Printed in Great Britain by St Edmundsbury Press Limited
Bury St Edmunds, Suffolk

Contents

General editor's introduction

My first meeting with Dr W. H. ('Bill') Mittins was at the very first annual conference of the National Association for the Teaching of English (NATE) in 1964 when he chaired the discussion group to which I was allocated. We have been firm friends ever since. He has also remained a valued and influential member of NATE, serving as Chairman, Secretary and Advisory Officer, probably the longest serving member of its Council and Executive.

For many years Bill was a lecturer in English education at the University of Newcastle upon Tyne. He was unusual in that his main interest in the field of English teaching was that of language, having written a grammar of modern English, done research into attitudes to English usage, and developed a particular expertise in semantics. In 1964 there were few people involved in educating young teachers of English who shared these interests and many of us were inclined to regard Bill as an amiable eccentric.

Now the wheel has turned full circle and language is very much in the consciousness of all of us. Sadly, it remains the case that it is only a minority of English studies at universities which involve any serious and systematic study of language but, subsequent to the Report of the Kingman Inquiry and that of the English Working Group on the National Curriculum, chaired by Professor Cox (both fully documented in this book), language is unmistakably on the agenda in the subject-English classroom.

Of course this was always the case elsewhere. It was significant that, at the first Anglo-American seminar on the teaching of English at Dartmouth, New Jersey, in 1966, most of the American participants took language very seriously. It was part of the 'trivium': language, literature and composition. Although there were a number of distinguished British linguists present, notably Professors Abercrombie and Sinclair (both, significantly, hailing from Edinburgh, not from an English university), most of the British contingent, including myself, had little interest in, and no knowledge of, the role of language in the classroom. Much later still, scholars like David Crystal were writing books with titles such as *What Is Linguistics?* It remained an arcane area of study.

So unfortunately it remains for many English teachers today. In spite of the demands of the National Curriculum, most university courses of English are unreconstructed, contrasting interestingly with those in polytechnics – literature still rules. There is, of course, no reason why we should object to the role of literature within the English curriculum; all one is arguing for is a little more balance so that more teachers of English go into their classrooms equipped with an understanding of modern approaches to language and with their minds cleared of the many myths about language – what has been called 'folklore linguistics' – that pass for knowledge in most cases.

Hence this book. When I invited Bill to write it I knew that what was needed was a clear introduction to language for the classroom teacher who had been through a conventional college or university English course, or, even more, for those many teaching English with, to quote the Bullock Report, 'no discernible qualification in the subject'. The Bullock Report, entitled *A Language For Life*, was perhaps the first official report to put language firmly in the forefront of the English curriculum. Since then there have been many others, including the now somewhat discredited HMI document, *English 5–16* (Curriculum Matters 1), which first introduced the idea of 'knowledge about language' into the curriculum. English teachers reacted against this with immediate vigour, often without having read the document at all carefully. For most any talk of 'language' was equated with a return to the formal teaching of traditional grammar which, for very good reasons, had been discounted in the immediate post-war period.

This was, in itself, an indication of the insecurity of many English teachers about the whole area of language study. Bullock had recommended whole-school policies for 'language across the curriculum'; mostly these failed because of the lack of both knowledge and will on the part of the teachers concerned. Gradually this term gave way to that of 'language awareness', a growing movement which sought to bring English teachers and teachers of other languages together in a common concern. Kingman and Cox have joined together in seeking to introduce 'knowledge about language' as a strand in the National Curriculum, though interestingly enough it still does not appear (at least as yet) as a separate attainment target. We have preferred here the terminology 'language awareness', both as being less threatening to those not already interested in this field and in its emphasis upon the unity of language concerns across subject boundaries.

Yet, for many teachers in Britain, language awareness remains something of which they are themselves largely unaware. What is needed is a clear, scholarly and readable introduction which will meet their felt need of a sound understanding of those areas of modern linguistic science which are relevant to the classroom and which have been absent from their own education. Indeed, with the decline of traditional grammar teaching since the 1950s, there is a whole generation of teachers of English to whom the whole field of language, even at the most elementary level, is a closed book.

Bill Mittins's book sets out to fill this gap. It has immense scholarship and a lifetime of work behind it, but it wears its scholarly mantle lightly. Not only is it eminently readable but it stands upon the assumption that language, as a primary human artefact, is uniquely fascinating as an object of study. Bill's own sense of excitement and fascination with his subject – and, as those who know him will readily recognize, of fun – is apparent on every page. It is, above all, 'a good read' as well as necessary reading for those struggling to equip themselves for the teaching of the new demands of the National Curriculum. To do this effectively will require knowledge; already there are language 'textbooks' being prepared that are old grammar books and gap-filling exercises writ anew. The present volume is as up to date as any book can be, given the inevitable time-lag between writing and production; it is a clear guide to the knowledge that is needed but, even more importantly, it leads its readers to understanding.

As an editor I am much indebted to Bill's painstaking and fascinating work.

Anthony Adams

Preface

John Trim, for many years Chairman of the Centre for Information on Language Learning and Research (CILT), once deplored (*Times Higher Education Supplement*, 28 March 1975, p. 18) the fact that 'the man in the street is better informed about nuclear physics, cosmology and genetics than about the language he [presumably also *she*] uses and hears all day and every day'. He observed that 'teachers, for whom language is the primary professional tool, and who consequently stand to gain most from a conscious awareness of its nature and use, too rarely have any opportunity for the systematic study of language in their academic education and professional training'. Consequently, he welcomed the work of Professor Sinclair and his collaborators on language in the classroom.

I have found John Sinclair's brief article on *Language Awareness in Six Easy Lessons* invaluable in providing a framework that imposes a measure of orderliness on what he calls the 'creative untidiness' of explorations into the many aspects of language. My sizeable bibliography in effect acknowledges debts to many other writers on language and languages. In particular, I am indebted to the work on discourse analysis done by Malcolm Coulthard (colleague of and collaborator with Sinclair) and to Geoffrey Leech's *Principles of Pragmatics*.

In the course of reading and quoting widely, I have been saddened to learn of the deaths of Peter Strevens and Paul Jennings. Both, in their very different ways, have attacked the notorious insularity of the English language. The end of the 1980s has also reminded us, through the televised reports of extraordinary events in Eastern Europe, how easy it is to recruit foreign speakers of English, and how difficult it is to find comparable British speakers of foreign languages.

W.H.M.

1 Language in the National Curriculum

'Sic biscuitus disintegrat' – That's the way the cookie crumbles.
(Iris Murdoch)

At the time of writing, the present government is poised between enacting a National Curriculum and implementing it. Only time can tell whether the legislation presided over by one Secretary of State for Education (Kenneth Baker) will be translated into effective action by his successor (John MacGregor). The new elaborate scheme is intended to set clear objectives, to check on performance at ages 7, 11, 14 and 16, to make schools – at least maintained schools in England and Wales – more accountable for the education they offer, and therefore to raise educational standards. The extent to which these intentions are realized must depend on how 'the cookie crumbles', that is, on how workable the scheme proves to be in actual teaching and testing practice. A recent article – 'Advisory body left out in the cold' (*Times Educational Supplement (TES)*, 3 November 1989) – suggests that the scheme is crumbling, if not collapsing. The School Examinations and Assessment Council (SEAC), it says, accuses government ministers of ignoring their advice by restricting both GCSE's coverage of the ability range and the use of records of achievement, and by reducing the role and status of teachers in assessing pupils at 7, 11 and 14 (see p. 18 below).

The Education Reform Act and school subjects

The 1988 Education Reform Act requires maintained schools to provide a balanced and broadly based curriculum comprising religious education and the National Curriculum. For law-making purposes a curriculum is regarded as a set of school 'subjects'. These subjects were once compared (by J. F. Kerr) with eggs in a crate, each fitting snugly into a pre-designed space, isolated from the rest. Some timetabled activities – in classrooms, laboratories, workshops, gymnasiums, on playing fields – accept the 'subject' designation fairly comfortably; others resist it. Her Majesty's Inspectorate (HMI) has admitted: 'When the curriculum is defined only in subjects, it is difficult to accommodate those aspects which tend to fall between the subject boundaries; for example, environmental education, economic awareness, and social education and new needs such as computer education' (Department of Education and Science (DES) 1985a, p. 10).

There are areas of language – specific foreign languages, formal grammar teaching, English literature – which fit more or less satisfactorily into the conventional scheme, but 'the linguistic talents a pupil possesses or can develop do not fall simply into the slots provided by school subject disciplines and are thus not the exclusive property of this or that department' (Robertson, 1980, p. 20). 'English' is the medium for all our teaching and operates across the curriculum. Moreover, English language is acquired before school age and its use is modified outside school. Again, the creative arts subjects might risk being squeezed out by the increased emphasis on traditional subjects. This possibility has elicited from the Minister of the Arts, Richard Luce, an inelegantly expressed – and not really convincing – assurance that the curriculum team for English would 'not only [consider] drama in the context of the great dramatic works of literature, but also as a medium for the development of a range of oral skills, which are relevant to all subjects'. He added that media studies would be considered (Lawlor, 1989).

Peter Strevens (1965, p. 74) gives English the most extensive coverage by suggesting that we 'agree to accept as "English" any piece of human behaviour that is clearly meaningful language, whether spoken or written, and which is not any language other than English'.

English in the National Curriculum

DES and Welsh Office (1987, p. 7) names 'English' as one of a score of subjects listed as 'foundation' or 'additional' components of the National Curriculum (NC). Elsewhere, stating that the legislation will not require particular subjects to be given specific *names* on school timetables, it accepts that labelling varies. The content and scope of most subjects – whether called, for instance, 'Home Economics' or 'Domestic Science', 'Business Studies' or 'Commercial Studies', 'Physical Training' or 'Physical Education' – are well enough understood to avoid serious differences. But because of the lack of consensus among teachers, 'English' notoriously presents problems of interpretation. Professor Cox, chairman of the English Working Group (EWG), believes that there has been a 'growing consensus' about what makes good English practice (*TES*, 25 November 1988), but Professor Rosen, addressing a conference at Nottingham University, is reported to have 'questioned whether the [Kingman] report's [DES, 1988] underlying assumption of a new consensus in English teaching was "possible" or desirable' (*TES*, 6 June 1988).

Ian Michael's (1987) detailed account of *The Teaching of English from the Sixteenth Century to 1870* ends with a chapter on 'English: the development of a subject'. In a section considering the term 'English', he refutes the common allegation that 'there was little or no teaching of English before the final decades of the nineteenth century.' Demonstrating that English was treated 'sometimes as a unity, sometimes as a blend of components', he compiles a tentative outline development of the subject in terms of its principal components:

From early times	Reading, spelling and pronunciation; some oral expression; perhaps some drama . . .
By 1525	Some written expression
By 1550	Some snatches of literature
By 1585	Grammar
By 1650	More substantial literature; more sustained written expression
By 1720	Some explicit teaching of literature; linguistic exercises in, or derived from, grammar and rhetoric
By 1730	Elocution
By 1750	More substantial dramatic work
By 1820	History of the language
By 1850	History of literature

(Michael, 1987, p. 381)

Later components would include elements of communication and media studies, of information technology, of unscripted 'creative' or 'educational' drama. Moreover, many teachers of native English (ENL) now need to deal with English as a second language (E2L) or as a foreign language (EFL) in order to meet the needs of 'immigrant' children. (We shall discuss multilingual and multicultural issues later in this chapter.) The broadest version of what may, *faute de mieux*, be referred to as an English-cum-Language course would include language-awareness matters spanning English and foreign languages. In contrast, the narrowest 'English' courses have focused more or less exclusively on particular segments of the subject. Over a long period, some teachers have chosen to treat either grammar or literature as sufficient for the teaching of English. Of language pedagogy before the nineteenth century it has been asserted, perhaps with some simplification, that 'grammar teaching was considered not only necessary but also sufficient. Until that time . . . language teaching and the study of grammar were virtually synonymous' (Rutherford and Smith, 1988, p. 9). On the other hand, a committee of teachers of English has argued – also with exaggeration – that 'Literature, the storehouse of recorded experiences, provides models for all the variety of uses to which we put language' (Incorporated Association of Assistant Masters, 1952). Both emphases have proved unsatisfactory. Grammar study can neglect the actual use of language. Others find literature insufficient, because of its concentration on work characteristically both written and commonly of an 'élitist' quality; moreover, they are not persuaded by more recent post-structuralist notions of 'textuality' that seem to extend 'literature' to include all stretches of language, irrespective of length and quality. Advocates of drama – both recorded text drama and improvised creative drama – with some justice make their specialism the focal point of English teaching. Increasingly, however, it seems implausible to regard English as a totally unitary subject; it must be accepted, in Michael's phrase, as a 'blend of components'.

Bullock

The Bullock Report broadened the notion of English teaching by choosing the title *A Language for Life* and by supporting the cause of 'language across the curriculum' (DES, 1975, Ch. 12). However, it restricted the latter cross-curricular concern to *English* language, justifying the exclusion of foreign languages from the committee's terms of reference. These terms asked for inquiry into 'all aspects of teaching the use of English'. Chapter 20 of the Report – on 'Children from Families of Overseas Origin' – briefly recognized the language problems of 'immigrant' children but, understandably, ruled it to be 'outside the scope of this Report to examine the advantages and disadvantages of the different types of provision made for teaching English as a second language'. It confined itself to admitting that systems offering specialist teaching (for example, in special centres), while often more practicable, suffered by isolating immigrant children and cutting them off 'from the social and educational life of a normal school' (para. 20.10).

Two examples of a Basic Language Course for teacher trainees are offered (para. 23.25). The first one begins by basing the study of 'the nature and function of language' on potential teachers' own language and on the language of school children. But, in the absence of indications to the contrary and given the monoglot character of the Report, the latter reference presumably means the language of native English-speaking children. Similarly, the 'Linguistic awareness and reading', mentioned in the same specification, doubtless means *English*-language awareness.

The Bullock Report broadened its brief from the intended initial focus on standards of reading English (specified by Secretary of State Margaret Thatcher), but felt bound to exclude English as a second language, thereby 'marginalizing' the needs of 'immigrant' children. Ten years later the Swann Report (DES 1985b) recognized these needs as central to 'Education for All'. It strengthened and amplified Bullock's doubts about 'isolating' systems using specialist centres. In a powerful paragraph on 'Language Awareness and Linguistic Diversity', it attacked excessive 'Anglicity':

> Within the concept of 'Education for All' there is also a need to broaden pupils' concept of language so that they no longer see it solely in terms of 'English', and come to appreciate the positive aspects of living in a linguistically diverse society. In a society in which the tradition of monolingualism is deeply entrenched and belief in the 'superiority' of the English language has been fostered by its historical relationship with the British Empire and its continuing role as a major international language, the concept of any other languages, even those of our European neighbours, as 'strange' and 'foreign' is perhaps understandable but hardly defensible. We should see the countering of such attitudes as an important component of 'education for all' and the heightening of all pupils' awareness of the range and richness of language as contributing to a better education for all. (DES, 1985b, p. 419)

After Bullock

The Bullock Report has been strongly criticized for its 'failure to allot any role in "language for life" to the study of foreign languages' and for perpetuating 'linguistic parochialism' by interpreting 'Across the curriculum' as not meaning 'across the *language* curriculum' and giving foreign-language teachers 'no role in it' (Hawkins, 1987, p. 27). If this was 'a great opportunity lost', the time has come to bring much closer together all the languages learned and used in Great Britain. During the past two decades or so, teachers of languages have combined to devise syllabuses which clarify what the nebulous phrase 'language awareness' can and should mean. The initiative has been taken in this by teachers of foreign languages and, in some cases, even by non-language teachers. Parallel to this work, the Kingman Inquiry and the English Working Group (EWG) have sought to establish a framework for the teaching of English as a core subject in the NC.

To what extent have relevant NC documents and the recommendations of 'English' committees been influenced by theoretical and practical work on the awareness of language? Have the two hitherto parallel routes converged? The languages and language-related subjects named in *The National Curriculum 5–16* (DES and Welsh Office, 1987) are:

English – a core foundation subject to be studied throughout schooling.
A modern foreign language – a foundation subject to be studied during the secondary phase.
Drama – one of four components making up a combined foundation subject for fourth- and fifth-year students.
A second modern foreign language, classics, drama – additional subjects.
Welsh – (i) a foundation subject in schools where Welsh is the teaching medium.
    – (ii) an available subject in English-speaking schools.
Technology – as far as it is relevant to language study, a foundation subject.

The DES has admitted that, while 'valuable progress has been made towards securing agreement about the objectives and content of particular subjects', such progress has been 'variable, uncertain and often slow'. To meet the government's wish 'to move ahead at a faster pace', it was assumed that 'a national curriculum *backed by clear assessment arrangements* will help to raise standards of attainment' (DES and Welsh Office, 1987, pp. 5, 6 and 8, emphasis added).

Task Group on Assessment and Testing

The terms of reference of the Task Group on Assessment and Testing (TGAT), set up in February 1987 and chaired by Professor Black, asked for advice, as stated in its report, on 'the practical considerations which should govern all assessment including testing of attainment at the ages of 7 (approximately), 11, 14 and 16, within a national curriculum' (DES and Welsh Office, 1988a, App. A).

Assessment and testing were obviously to be an essential part of educational reform.

Before considering TGAT's impact on languages in general, it is necessary to note the awkwardness – presumably serving 'faster pace' – which established, also 'at the beginning of 1987', the Committee of Inquiry into the Teaching of English Language. The two committees doubtless recognized the need to collaborate, but it was not until 30 October 1987 that Professor Black officially received advice from Elizabeth House that his Group 'will need to liaise closely . . . with the Committee on English chaired by Sir John Kingman'. Partly because the TGAT Report was published as early as December 1987, some months before (in March 1988) the Kingman Report (DES, 1988a) appeared, there is reason to doubt whether the liaison was either close or frequent. It is not surprising that, compared with its treatment of mathematics and science – the other core subjects – TGAT has rather less to say about English or indeed about language in general.

Teachers of 'subject-English' may be less impressed than colleagues teaching foreign languages that 'when assessment and testing are carefully aligned to the curriculum, as in *Graded Assessment Schemes*, one of the outstanding benefits that teachers report is the enhanced motivation of pupils' (DES and Welsh Office 1988a, para. 14, emphasis added). The notion of 'graded assessment' seems to reinforce an assumption that a mother-tongue language can be taught and assessed with as much linear progressiveness or staging as has proved successful with foreign languages. Underlying this notion is the questionable assumption of 'successivity' which dominates the secondary school curriculum and indeed 'runs right through British academic life. Successful study of most subjects at a given level, it is assumed, rests on successful study of that subject (or a different but relevant one) at the previous one' (Pearce, 1972, pp. 89–90). It smacks further of the broader and dubious theory that everything that exists must exist in some degree and therefore be measurable. These assumptions are explicitly challenged by the insistence in the Cox EWG Reports (DES and Welsh Office, 1988b; 1989) on the 'recursive', 'iterative' and 'non-linear' character of native language learning.

Appendix C of the TGAT Report records Meetings with Invited Groups. The 'teams' of the Assessment of Performance Unit submitted materials used in schemes both for well-defined subjects (including Foreign Languages) and for relatively undefined 'Language'. A previous paragraph (DES and Welsh Office, 1988a, App. C, para. 1) dealing with graded assessment, records meetings, among others, with representatives of the Joint Matriculation Board's Staged Assessment in Literacy. TGAT accepts that literacy 'has applications well beyond what might be contained within English' (DES and Welsh Office, 1988a, para. 143). An 'announcement on assessment' made by the Secretary of State, at that time Kenneth Baker, is printed as Appendix 4 to the second Cox Report on *English for ages 5 to 16* (DES and Welsh Office, 1989). There, 'English' – specifically so named – is aligned with the other major subjects. The expressed expectation is that the principles established by TGAT would 'inform the consultations which will take place later this year [1989] on the recommendations of the National Curriculum Mathematics and Science Working Groups, and likewise [to] inform the thinking of the Working Groups on English and Design and Technology which we announced last month'.) Appendix C of the TGAT report (DES and Welsh Office, 1988a) adds that 'Developing practice in graded assessment in modern [foreign] languages was also considered.' Earlier, discussing profile components, it associates schemes in English that 'attend separately to writing, oracy, reading comprehension, and listening' with, 'similarly', the three components that contribute to graded assessments in science developed with the London Group (DES and Welsh Office, 1988a, para. 33). The first Cox Report, recognizing the four aspects mentioned by TGAT, was to emphasize that 'development in the four language modes is complex and *non-linear*' (DES and Welsh Office, 1988b, para. 1.8, emphasis added). Pam Czerniewska points out that the non-linear character of first-language learning had been demonstrated earlier – in the Inspectorate's *English from 5 to 16* – by the repetitiveness of age-related objectives specified as

> for 7-year-olds: Set down directions and instructions when there is a clear purpose
> for doing so
> for 11-year-olds: Frame instructions and directions clearly
> for 16-year-olds: Frame instructions and directions clearly and succinctly
>
> (Czerniewska, 1988, p. 125)

(The implications seem to be: at age 7, the purpose but not necessarily the writing needs to be clear; at age 11, be clear, but not necessarily succinct; at age 16, be both!)

The possible difficulty of reconciling non-linearity of the subject with graded assessment of achievement in it was not examined by TGAT, presumably because incompatibility between the two might have threatened the assumptions about assessment underlying the whole National Curriculum.

A similar difficulty, also to be tackled when the assessment system comes into operation, is presented by the 'shift from norm-referencing to criterion-referencing' (DES and Welsh Office, 1988a, para. 7). Though criterion-referencing is allegedly interpreted with 'a broader and less exacting definition than that used by some authors', it still seeks – as norm-referencing does not – to make judgments of what in the Glossary is defined as 'the absolute quality of the performance'. (This appeal to *absolute quality* seems diametrically opposed, at least in language teaching, to Sapir's (1924, p. 157) more persuasive view that 'It is the appreciation of the relativity of the form of thought which results from linguistic study that is perhaps the most liberalizing thing about it. What fetters the mind and benumbs the spirit is ever the dogged acceptance of absolutes'.) Subject-English has notoriously been afflicted by problems of achieving both high reliability and high validity. Many years ago (1924), William Boyd's investigation of measurement in composition and spelling (as well as arithmetic) demonstrated how inflated weighting of 'objective' qualities (such as spelling, 'absence-of-mistakes', frequency of unique or unusual words) could achieve very high reliability in marking at the expense of validity, that is, of measuring what purports to be measured. Obviously, English composition is more than a matter of readily countable features. 'Absence of mistakes' is a meanly negative criterion for assessing quality. TGAT's Appendix G concludes dauntingly that 'Users cannot be expected to be familiar with the translation of reliability or validity indices into confidence limits' and suggests (unrealistically because expensively?) that the necessary analysis 'will have to be undertaken by expert agencies'.

Both gender and ethnic bias affect assessment of language performance. They are briefly considered together as forms of invalidity in two paragraphs (DES and Welsh Office, 1988a, paras 51–2). The recommendation is that 'assessment tasks be reviewed regularly for evidence of bias, particularly in respect of gender and race'. Having collected the evidence, 'as far as possible the sources of such bias should be eliminated'. This somewhat vague expression of hope is presumably given some substance in a submission by the Equal Opportunities Commission (EOC) reproduced as Appendix F to TGAT. The EOC accepts that complete elimination of gender bias in test construction is as yet unlikely to be achieved, and therefore 'a complicated statistical adjustment would be necessary' – presumably also to be conducted by 'expert agencies'.

For the language handicaps of those whose first language is not English, TGAT – again briefly and without going into practical implications – recognizes that a pupil's low level of performance merely indicates that he or she needs 'special help in English language skills' and suggests that 'assessment in other skills and understanding, particularly at age 7, should, wherever practicable and necessary, be conducted in the pupil's first language' (DES and Welsh Office, 1988a, para. 53). The remarkable rapidity with which TGAT produced a novel assessment procedure probably made it inevitable that some important but not central matters of concern are treated rather cursorily, relying sometimes on appendices to tackle details. According to a *TES* report (10 March 1989), Professor Nuttall expressed pessimistic views about the future of TGAT, mainly but not solely because of its failure to deal satisfactorily with bilingualism. He thought that it is 'completely impractical' to apply the tests through the very many languages – 170 alone in the Inner London Education Authority (ILEA) area. He doubted whether 'tests can be translated into other languages'. The 'vision' of Professor Black had become 'distorted' because teacher assessment and moderation were being 'pushed further down the agenda' and because tests would fail to eliminate bias or to achieve validity and comparability. Consequently, 'the SAT [Standard Assessment Task] programme might ring its own death knell' and the government should therefore scrap what Nuttall says has become a 'monster of an external system'.

Examples of the variety of forms of assessment available are given in DES (1988b, App. E). In all the 21 examples used, the stated 'task mode', 'response mode' or 'presentation mode' (or two or three of these) is partly or wholly linguistic, oral or written. Two examples (nos 15 and 18) test modern foreign languages, respectively German and French. The five native-language tests (nos 10–14) focus on the skills of literacy and oracy rather than more generally on English language and literature as usually understood.

Kingman

In Britain, or at least in British schools, language awareness means awareness of the many languages used in our schools. The list includes first languages, second languages and foreign languages. Of the thousands of possible tongues, the Kingman Report refers primarily, of course, to English as a first language. It also briefly mentions:

1 English as a second or foreign language
2 Welsh and Gaelic as first languages
3 French, Latin and Punjabi as foreign languages taught in British schools
4 Polish, Ukrainian, Urdu, Gujarati, Cantonese, Turkish, and
5 Afro-Caribbean Creole, Japanese, Brazilian and Russian accents in speaking English.

These references are in the main incidental and auxiliary to mother-tongue English. The convenient, perhaps necessary, notion of separate school subjects supports the concept of 'mother tongues' which are clearly separable from 'foreign' languages. A less convenient, less manageable notion is that based on Bakhtin's (1981) distinction between two opposing forces operating in all language. In the interpretation of his argument offered by Hopkins (1989, pp. 200–1), 'heteroglossia' (the coexistence of dialects in language) contrasts with 'polyglossia' (the coexistence of fragments of several 'foreign' languages within every 'mother tongue'). Consequently, 'the concept of a "pure" language is a delusion'. The circumstances in which the Kingman Inquiry was set up virtually induced it to adopt a strategy assuming that the English language could be treated, if not as 'pure', then as separable enough for it to be given priority over 'foreign' languages. The subsequent governmental regulation (see p. 17) produced the invidious 'league table' division into two foreign language groups – on the one hand, modern European foreign languages specified in the National Curriculum, on the other (by implication less important) hand, non-European Community languages.

Less peripheral are proposals of closer collaboration between teachers of English and teachers of modern European foreign languages. The chapter on teacher training finds 'merit in the suggestion that students of English and of modern languages [English does not count as a *modern* language for this purpose!] should, wherever possible, work together in planning and delivering a "language-focussed" project to a shared class of pupils' (DES, 1988, para. 6.6).

In dealing with 'Co-ordinating language study in schools', the Report (DES, 1988, para. 4.50) notes that 'In many schools in England "language awareness courses" of different kinds are being taught'. It adds somewhat ambivalently that these courses 'vary in quality'. It applauds the 'enthusiastic openness to language study' shown by some (by implication, not all) such courses. It goes on to observe, rather vaguely, that these things can ensure that all teachers of language in a school use 'the same framework of description for talking about language' with 'the same descriptive vocabulary'. The problem of establishing a common terminology is more difficult than the need for a common descriptive terminology allows. Professor Sonnenschein and the Joint Committee on Grammatical Terminology failed as long ago as 1909 to devise a nomenclature acceptable to teachers of the various school languages.

A related but more important aspect of English-language teaching has been the advocacy of 'language across the curriculum' (l.a.c.). The movement favouring this development was launched by *Language, the learner and the school* (Barnes *et al.*, 1969). Harold Rosen's contribution, on behalf of the London Association for the Teaching of English (LATE), was a discussion document on 'Towards a Language Policy Across the Curriculum'. Appearing as Part III, it followed pieces – by Douglas Barnes and James Britton – on language in learning. The l.a.c. arguments were endorsed by the Bullock committee as wanting closer collaboration among most school subjects, though, as we have already noticed, it did not include modern foreign languages. Even so, l.a.c. – despite the restricted Bullock interpretation – broadens the understanding of 'English' and therefore takes a step towards Anglocentric, if not universal, 'language awareness'.

The actual references to l.a.c. in the Kingman Report are cryptic. To comment that the phrase 'language across the curriculum' has been 'assimilated into educational jargon' (DES, 1988, para. 2.28) has a questionable connotation. It is only compatible with recognition of the importance of l.a.c. if one accepts that 'the notion was widely misinterpreted in the years after Bullock' (DES, 1988, para. 6.8). The Kingman document's stylistic addiction to academic litotes ('we have *no* doubt that . . .', 'it is *not* necessary to . . .', 'there is *no* reason why the subject of the English language should *not* be discussed . . .') warily claims that 'this is *not* to dismiss' the importance of l.a.c. but leaves the wide misinterpretation unexplored except for a parenthesized invitation to 'see *Bullock Revisited*'. This pamphlet, published in 1982 and ending deprecatingly with a couple of pages on 'what it [the Bullock Report] called "language across the curriculum"', suggests that the strategy of 'a policy "embedded in the organisational structure of the school", desirable as it is, may have been seen by some teachers as a requirement to adapt themselves to a theory derived from a subject discipline other than their own.' While l.a.c. was rated as probably the 'most widely noted message received from Bullock' and while 'many LEAs have actively encouraged secondary schools to develop such a policy', it was found that 'only a minority of schools have been able to translate such a policy into effective practice'. In all probability revealing the origin of the 'not widely understood' judgment, the pamphlet quotes from the Inspectorate's *Aspects of Secondary Education* (1979) that:

> it may be, indeed, that the phrase [l.a.c.] itself had not been widely enough understood or that it is not forceful enough to convey the notion of overall responsibility of all teachers for the development of language essential to learning . . .
>   In a great majority of schools throughout the three years of the [*Aspects*] survey, no moves of any significance have taken place . . .
>
> (DES, 1979, 6.6, 1–2)

Obviously l.a.c., like any other cross-curricular innovation, challenges the entrenched subject-based curriculum and the 'touch-me-not' defensive attitude of teacher specialists towards their own specialisms. Michael Marland, recognizing (1980) that 'the call for "across the curriculum" planning runs counter to the vertical, separate-subject tradition of syllabus planning', sees Irene Robertson's project as revealing the nature of the problems and says that it 'describes vividly the complexity of the tension between autonomy and coherence in our schools' (Robertson, 1980, p. 7). Her Majesty's Inspectors seem to resort to a pussy-footed pirouetting round the edges of these problems rather than directly confronting them. In this, their delicacy contrasts sharply with the more brutal seizure of the total curriculum (and, indeed, the teaching profession) by the recent Secretary of State for Education, Kenneth Baker.

In the event, the Kingman working party might appropriately have reduced the title of its report from the very broad 'Inquiry into the teaching of the English language' by adding a qualifying phrase or sub-title limiting it to 'Certain aspects of . . .' or 'A Model for . . .'. A more modest claim would have helped justify the remarkable shortness of the report and its sizeable omissions. It might then have been able to refute accusations that it 'failed to mention the Swann Report and seriously neglected the role of linguistic diversity in teaching English' (*TES*, 24 June 1988, reporting Rosen's address to the Nottingham conference).

The Kingman Committee accepted the emphasis in its terms of reference on designing a 'model' and specifying what pupils might be expected to understand about language at ages 7, 11 and 16 (age 14 was, curiously, not specified). Though it sought, as its Secretary said, 'to combine two streams of thought – of sociologists who said language teaching should be related to learning generally and of those who called for a more structured approach', it veered noticeably towards the latter. This favoured the assumption, adopted by most professional linguists and by the scientifically-minded, that language is well-defined. The other 'stream of thought', preferred by many teachers and more sympathetic to language awareness, accepts the more intractable, less tidy character of language. It is significant that at least one reputable linguist – the American Charles Hockett (1967, pp. 61–2) – has admitted moving from a more rigorous position to a more tolerant, more 'teacher-friendly' acceptance of comparative untidiness:

I now believe that any approximation we can achieve on the assumption that language is well-defined is obtained by leaving out of account just those properties of real language that are most important. For at bottom the productivity and power of language – our casual ability to say new things – would seem to stem exactly from the fact that languages are not well-defined, but merely characterized by certain degrees and kinds of *stability*.

The Inquiry 'sets the scene' in its Chapter 1, which makes no reference to non-English languages except for deploring the 'inadequate account of the English language by treating it [as old-fashioned grammar teaching does] as a branch of Latin' (DES, 1988, para. 1.11). (In this, they were – knowingly or otherwise – following a precedent set three centuries ago by Joseph Aickin (1693), who had challenged slavish adherence to the Latin model by writing *The English grammar, or the English tongue reduced to grammatical rules . . . In learning whereof the English scholar may now obtain the perfection of his mother tongue, without the assistance of Latin.* They were also implying that the American Mencken (1936, p. 52) was being unduly optimistic or flattering in claiming in 1919 that 'the English themselves' had *long since* abandoned the notion that English grammar was a kind of Latin grammar and that 'English [British?] teachers of English were therefore required to inculcate grammatical niceties'.) Exclusive 'Anglicity' is maintained throughout Chapter 2, dealing with the importance of knowledge about language. This chapter ends with the reasonable affirmation that 'The word "language" is an abstraction; it subsumes all the reasons by which human beings communicate . . . with each other'. But 'any model of language must be, to a greater or lesser extent, *specific*' (DES, 1988, para. 2.39). It could be argued that learning about how language works, though made tidier by confinement to a single language, could be made more informative, more interesting and less 'parochial' by cross-referencing to other languages. And, of course, multilingual approaches should be helpful to multiracial classes.

The actual model presented in Chapter 3, accepting the Inquiry's Anglocentric terms of reference, proceeds from initial examination of 'The forms of the English language', through communication, comprehension, acquisition and development, to historical and geographical variation. In the fold-out summary of the model (DES, 1988, Appendix 8) there are no references to languages other than English except in the very last Figure 5, where language changes are said to 'mark different dialects (*or eventually different languages*)' (emphasis added). Chapter 4, discussing 'the model in use' has a general recommendation (DES, 1988, para. 4.33) on the need for teachers 'to instil in their pupils a civilised respect for other languages and an understanding of the relations between other languages and English'. Among the examples of class-room good practice, one illustration describes a lesson in which a fairy-tale read to 7-year-olds mostly of Asian parentage led to finding lists of words of similar and then of opposite meaning in English and Urdu (DES, 1988, para. 4.35). Further bilingual examples, suitable for older children and exploring more extensive language features (for example, sentence structures, discourse procedures) would have helped usefully to moderate the monolinguistic emphasis on English.

From Kingman to the English Working Group

The Kingman Inquiry was sandwiched between *earlier* official pressure and the promise of a *later* EWG. The EWG produced two reports (DES and Welsh Office, 1988b; 1989), each being printed in a document labelled 'Proposals of the Secretaries of State for Education (in England and Wales)'. The later report includes the substance and often the wording of the earlier.

The EWG was required 'to build on the recommendations of the Kingman Report with respect to children's knowledge of "the grammatical structure of the English language", and more generally with respect to "children's explicit and implicit knowledge about language"' (DES and Welsh Office, 1988b, para. 5.1). By gearing the EWG to the Kingman model, 'knowledge about language' preserves the primacy of language-specific English over language universals. Presumably it was because Professor Widdowson, as a member of the Kingman Committee, accepted the English-specific limitations imposed upon it, that he does not refer in his 'Note of reservation' (DES 1988, App. 3) to the Teaching of English to Speakers of Other Languages (TESOL), even though he himself heads a TESOL Department in the London University Institute of Education. Nevertheless, his regret that the Kingman model 'does not come to grips with the central question of . . . what English is on the curriculum *for*' must surely bear on the needs – especially in London – of pupils with first languages other than English. Professor Brumfit (1988) thinks that the Kingman terms of reference 'could easily have been modified to recognize the indivisibility of language acquisition in a multicultural society'.

Widdowson refers to the 'seven brief paragraphs covering the complexities of adult uses of language'. With tantalizing brevity, these paragraphs mention language features ranging from the philosophical – 'Language is the naming of experiences and what we name we have power over', 'People need expertise in language to be able to participate effectively in a democracy' – to humdrum matters of the 'carpentry of life', such as form-filling, job competence and family relationships. Cutting across all these language roles is the fact of change, of accelerated change including linguistic change. All these generalizations are anything but English-specific. They have important implications for an increasingly multicultural society such as Britain's. This fact is recognized by the official supplementary guidance asking the EWG 'to take account of the ethnic diversity of the school population and society at large, bearing in mind the cardinal point that English shall be the first language and medium of instruction for all pupils in England' (DES and Welsh Office, 1989, para. 10.1, and App. 3, para. 13). The Committee for Linguistics in Education (CLIE) urged that explicit consideration of the language of ethnic minorities could 'raise the social status of the languages themselves' (CLIE, 1984, p. 9). Katharine Perera, who was to become a very active member of the EWG, endorses this view, adding that 'The study of some of the differences within and between languages is one way in which the ideals of multi-culturalism could become a living reality in the classroom' (Perera, 1987, p. 17).

The Kingman Committee was appointed by the DES, but the EWG was made responsible also to the Secretary of State for Wales. It is not surprising, therefore, that the Cox terms of reference required advice on a framework which would 'ensure, at the minimum, that all school-leavers are competent in the use of English – written and spoken – *whether or not it is their first language*' (DES and Welsh Office, 1988b, App. 2; 1989, para. 10.1, emphasis added). The Kingman Inquiry addressed in particular English *language*, and took this to mean primarily the forms and structures of the native language. The Cox group, being an *English* working party, was able to range more widely. Under the heading of 'Historical and geographical variation' and in a context contrasting Standard English with dialects, the Kingman Report included a statement about other languages than English. It added that those

> knowledgeable about the process of language change, and in particular the history of English, can reflect and comment illuminatingly on such matters as . . . the ways in which, historically and currently, groups settling in Britain have enriched English (and created a multi-lingual community in which many languages other than English, Welsh and Gaelic now subsist side by side – Polish, Ukrainian, Urdu, Gujarati, Afro-Caribbean creole languages, Cantonese, Turkish, and so on). (DES, 1988a, para. 3.20)

Ethnic-minority languages are neither included as subjects (not even 'additional' subjects) in the National Curriculum nor given (as they might conceivably have been) a status analogous to the 'Special Position of Welsh'. But they are sensibly linked in the Cox reports with the European languages taught in schools. Cox insists not only that 'the curriculum for all pupils should include informed discussion of the multi-cultural nature of British society, whether or not the individual school is culturally mixed', but also that

> the development of competence in spoken and written Standard English is sensitive to the knowledge of other languages which many children have. As well as the many different mother tongues that are present in our multi-cultural, multi-lingual society, there are also the foreign languages that are taught in schools. A rich source of insight into the nature of language is lost if English is treated in complete isolation. (DES and Welsh Office, 1988b, para. 3.7; 1989, para. 2.8)

Not as attainment targets but as aims of education to which English contributes, children at school-leaving stage should have acquired, among other things and as far as possible, 'an awareness of some of the properties of human languages and their role in societies' (DES and Welsh Office, 1988b, para. 3.11; 1989, para. 2.12). These arguments clearly support in principle the purposes of the 'language awareness' movement, though they do not, of course, endorse any of the particular language awareness programmes followed in diverse schools.

With its concern extending into the secondary years, the second Cox report obviously has more to say on 'Knowledge about language' (on which it has a full chapter), especially as far as it can be treated systematically. The 'richer and broader work' observed in some of the multilingual classrooms visited is approved for providing awareness of 'some of the similarities and differences among their [the pupils'] languages' (DES and Welsh Office, 1989, para 6.3). One of the 'helpful distinctions' that can be made in studying language is that between monolingual and bilingual competence (DES and Welsh Office, 1989, para. 6.10; cf. 1988b, para. 12.9) explicitly using the 'huge resources' provided by the many pupils who 'are bilingual and sometimes biliterate, and quite literally know more about language than their teachers, at least in some respects' (DES and Welsh Office, 1989, para. 6.11). Social benefits would clearly accrue from 'more understanding of language diversity, including multilingualism' (para. 6.14). Much research seems to support this view. The alleged drawbacks of 'cognitive overload' and relative lack of fluency in both (or more) languages are probably outweighed by benefits. George Saunders (1983, pp. 17–20) has summarized the advantages that bilingual compared with monolingual children can enjoy. These, which he describes in more detail, are:

Earlier and greater awareness of the arbitrariness of language
Earlier separation of meaning from sound
Greater adeptness at evaluating non-empirical contradictory statements
Greater adeptness at divergent thinking
Greater adeptness at creative thinking
Greater social sensitivity
Greater facility in concept formation.

English is a dominant, an increasingly dominant, world language. Crystal (1987b, p. 358) reports 'conservative estimates' that it is used as a mother tongue by 300 million speakers, as a second language by a further 300 million, as a foreign language by another 100 million. Moreover, the English language has been more thoroughly studied than most other languages. But these facts do not necessarily make English representative of all languages. In some ways, in fact, English is not a typical language. Aitchison (1987, p. 205) points out that – untypically – a large proportion of English speakers are literate and 'many English speakers are monolingual, a situation somewhat unusual in the world at large, where it is common for humans to use more than one language'. The Anglocentric bias suggested by these circumstances supports arguments for a measure of bilingualism. It makes particularly relevant the 'Special Position of Welsh', which is dealt with briefly in the second Cox report, Chapters 10 and 13 and in greater detail in the report of the Welsh Working Group (WWG) on *Welsh for ages 5 to 16* (Welsh Office, 1989).

As a contribution to acquiring knowledge about language, 'the bilingualism of Wales can be used to positive advantage to inform learning about language . . . The growth of confidence in two languages – English and Welsh – can only enhance insight into how language works' (Welsh Office, 1989, para. 2.17). Obviously, in broader contexts, the English-Welsh pairing can be matched – variously according to needs and resources – by other pairs of languages. Arguments that the 'comparative study of different languages' is for children a utopian waste of time (Knight, 1989, p. 21) and that 'bilingual education adversely affects skill in English or general conceptual understanding' are rejected. Unpublished Welsh research had found that the performance of bilingual 7-year-olds compared favourably with that of monolingual pupils. Moreover, an investigation undertaken by the English-based National Foundation for Educational Research (NFER) had shown that 'the English of pupils educated bilingually is at least equivalent to that of pupils taught through the medium of English' (Welsh Office, 1989, para. 2.23). In a chapter entitled 'Language Issues', the WWG Report repeatedly refers to 'awareness', emphasizing – in relation to Welsh, but presumably to all language teaching – that 'encouraging awareness and understanding of language can lead to improved mastery of it' (para. 5.2). Among the linguistic features mentioned as illuminating contrasts between Welsh and English are 'the flexibility of word order in Welsh sentences' (para. 5.20), the use of the 'long forms' of a verb in relative or adjectival clauses as against the apparently more sophisticated 'short forms' in relative clauses (para. 10.15), and the process of 'mutation' by which apparently consonants may change at the beginnings of words (para. 10.36).

Compared with the Welsh Working Group, the EWG was in the favourable position of concentrating on the teaching of the quantitatively major language, English, which 'is the first language of five out of six pupils in Wales and is the main medium of instruction in the great majority of schools' (DES and Welsh Office, 1989, para. 13.1). It is reported, indeed, that 11 English-speaking Welsh schools have already gone so far as to ask to be exempt from having to teach Welsh as a foundation subject. On the other hand, the WWG, aiming at raising the linguistic status of Welsh, was convinced by the qualitative cultural value of the language and of the consequent need to promote it both as a first and as a second language. Encouraged by 'the great steps taken to extend Welsh as a medium in the increasing number of primary and secondary schools in both Welsh-speaking and non-Welsh-speaking areas, and the accompanying increase in the provision of resources' (Welsh Office, 1989, para. 7.1), they devote a sizeable chapter to 'Welsh across the Curriculum'. There they embrace enthusiastically and optimistically the 'new areas' of dramatic role-play, electronic media and computers. As methods of making language learning 'as natural, amusing and painless as possible', and especially for presenting Welsh as a second language, they advocate the use of videos and computers. Many of the Programmes of Study for second-language Welsh specify activities such as playing computer games, using electronic mail, and using word processors and desktop publishing packages. The feasibility and possible success of these methods in facilitating the acquisition of Welsh as a second language could affect practice, not only in the teaching of first-language English, but in teaching foreign languages and in developing bilingualism (or multilingualism) among speakers of ethnic minority languages.

Other languages

Chapter 10 of the second Cox report looks more specifically at the position of bilingual children. Evidence suggests that 'some 5% of all schools in England are likely to have a significant population of children for whom English is not their mother tongue' (DES and Welsh Office, 1989, para. 10.3). The EWG links the English needs of this minority with the 'very great pool of linguistic competence' which they make available to the foreign language needs of English pupils. The Minister of State for Education (Angela Rumbold) has, in bland official phraseology, judged that circumstances offer 'a considerable challenge to us all to develop international understanding, a heightened awareness of Europe and, above all, a greater speed and proficiency in our foreign language learning' (*DES News*, 31/89, 31 January 1989). Later, announcing the constitution of the Modern Foreign Languages Working Group, she has reminded us that a modern foreign language is a foundation subject in the National Curriculum. This represents 'a very major change'. Despite Dr Johnson's contentious warning that 'Commerce, however necessary, however lucrative, as it depraves the manners, corrupts the language', the present government treats language – and many other affairs – in a commercially minded fashion. For Mrs Rumbold, 'the challenge of 1992 makes it imperative that we are prepared linguistically for the Single Market'. To meet this challenge (one hopes, for educational and social as well as commercial reasons), the 50 per cent of pupils who do not at present take a modern foreign language at age 15 or 16 will join the other half. The Supplementary Guidance to the new Working Group says that studying a modern foreign language should, among other things, offer pupils insight into the structure of language and of language learning (*DES News*, 261/89, 15 August 1989). This coincides so exactly with one of the objectives of English language learning that the sharing of teaching between teachers of English and of foreign languages in a language-awareness enterprise would seem logical as well as economical.

As yet, modern foreign languages are the European ones traditionally taught in our schools. Answering a Parliamentary Question and confirming a Statutory Instrument, the Secretary of State (then Kenneth Baker) said that he proposed two groups of languages for study. The first set are the 'working languages of the European Community', a list which includes modern Greek and Portuguese but not Irish. The second (non-EC) set are named as Arabic, Bengali, Gujarati, Hindi, Japanese, Mandarin and Cantonese Chinese, Punjabi, Turkish and Urdu. 'Maintained schools will be allowed, but not required, to offer one or more of these, in addition to those in the first group, as the National Curriculum modern foreign language' (*DES News* 66/89, 3 March 1989). One expert has accused the government of being 'crassly insensitive' by creating what will inevitably become first and second division league tables. This has been done, characteristically, *before* appointing the relevant working group and asking it whether it agrees with the decision. However, perhaps because of a political reshuffle involving a change of Secretary of State for Education, the dual division may, as suggested by ministerial guidance, be overruled. Whatever happens, the complexity of the languages scene emphasizes the importance of language awareness as a major factor in language affairs.

Interim stock-taking

It is far too soon after the actual launching of the National Curriculum to venture anything but the most tentative judgment of its prospective success or failure. The most dramatic pronouncement so far has been the strongly expressed view of Professor Nuttall (ILEA's director of research and statistics). Whatever the virtues of the TGAT proposals, he is sure that they will be so 'distorted' by the first trials of the prescribed national tests as to sound the 'death knell' of the SAT programmes that are central to what has become a 'monster of an external assessment system' (see page 8). This verdict looks at best premature, but it strengthens worries about the large role assigned to assessment and tests. Peter Newsam (1989) appears to foresee a procedure – perversely borrowed from the USA – in which 'both teachers and pupils, in the name of accountability, are tested to the edge of destruction'. Already there are indications – from reports of the SEAC deliberations – that the TGAT recommendation that assessment should include a teacher-assessment component is being rejected, at least partially, in order to give national external tests a decisive overriding authority. SEAC supported TGAT's recommendation on the role of teachers in assessment at 7, 11 and 14, but apparently it expressed the sensible view that it is essential 'to keep the demands made upon teachers' time . . . within acceptable limits'. According to an *Observer* report (22 October 1989), this led to the administratively convenient conclusion that 'the standard assessment procedures should take "preference" over teachers' ratings'. The elasticity of 'acceptable limits' and degrees of 'preference' permitted the Minister of State's decision to reduce the assessing role of teachers ostensibly so as not to 'add to the volume of work already undertaken by schools'. Such decisions – as reported in the *TES* of 3 November 1989 (see above, page 1) – left SEAC 'out in the cold' by ruling that, instead of allowing GCSE results to apply to the full ability-range of 16-year-olds (as recommended by SEAC), lower grades should count as failures, and that the widest use of records of achievement (recommended by SEAC) should not cover more than national curriculum assessment.

Behind these restrictions it is possible to detect intervention by the Prime Minister, who, again according to the *Observer* writer (interestingly surnamed 'Tester'), seemed to have overruled Kenneth Baker, as well as appointed experts, in 'insisting that children are rated according to nationally prescribed tests rather than by their teachers', because the judgements of the latter 'might be biased and untrustworthy'. In any case the TGAT blueprint 'would be too complex and expensive to introduce'.

The two Cox reports emphasize the non-linear character of language learning. Cox 1 (DES and Welsh Office, 1988b, para. 1.8) states that 'in formulating our recommendations we have taken heed of the point that development in the four language modes is complex and non-linear'. Then the final chapter of Cox 2 on Assessment (repeating DES and Welsh Office, 1988b, para. 7.5) acknowledges 'the problems in defining a linear sequence of language development'. Basing its observation on the findings of a great deal of research, it firmly states that 'children do not learn particular features of written language, for example, once and for all at any particular stage; they continually return to the same features and refine their competence' (DES and Welsh Office, 1989, para. 14.5). This is as familiar to many teachers of English language as the fact that the example from writing also applies to the other language modes.

Exponents of language-awareness theories extend these criticisms to cover the insufficient treatment of foreign-language contributions to the understanding of language in general. Collaboration among teachers of languages could help eradicate what Whitehead (1932, p. 10) has described as 'the fatal disconnection of subjects which kills the vitality of our modern curriculum'. Against these alleged inadequacies can be set opinions that the Cox reports have moved admirably in the direction of broadening conceptions of English, particularly by emphasizing the centrality of talk and endorsing much of present good English-teaching practice. The EWG reports have been described as 'surprisingly liberal'. Official committee work cannot realistically be expected to generate ecstasy, but, even so, it is a mark of considerable favour that the recommendations have been accepted with 'relief but little rapture'. This relief was mainly for the firm dismissal – by Kingman as well as Cox – of the dreaded retreat to traditional grammar. It was apparently more a concern to get publicity that led the Business in the Community (BiC) agency to invite newspaper reporters to attend an informal meeting of a handful of senior executives to be addressed by the BiC's president, Prince Charles. His off-the-cuff remarks, especially that 'English is taught so bloody badly' and that proper education is impossible without 'a basic framework and drilling system', certainly got plenty of publicity. His drilling system was assumed – for example, by the *TES* reporter – to be 'the traditional formal parsing [whatever that is] which the report rejects'. The expulsion of traditional Latinate grammar has often been accused of sacrificing the bath as well as the bathwater.

The twentieth century has seen repeated investigations, on both sides of the Atlantic, demonstrating that the teaching of formal, Latin-based, pre-linguistic traditional grammar has had no beneficial results. Professor Wilkinson has summarized the results of this research. They include findings that 'Training in formal grammar does not improve pupils' composition', that 'A knowledge of grammar is of no general help in correcting faulty usage', that 'Grammar may in fact hinder children's use of English', and that 'Grammar is often taught to children who have not the maturity in intelligence to understand it' (Wilkinson, 1971, pp. 33–4). Much of this research is decisive – but within limits. It applies only to traditional grammar and hardly justifies Wilkinson's judgement that 'it seems unlikely that the results would prove different with any of the new grammars'. The Scottish empirical investigation by Macauley into 'The Difficulty of Grammar' (claiming to validate the last of the above conclusions), for instance, was based on the measurement of schoolboys' success or failure in identifying some (not all) parts of speech as isolated items in short sentences and not as elements making up grammatical patterns (see Mittins, 1988, pp. 69–72). The Macauley investigation may, as suggested by Hunter Diack (1955), show 'no more than it is not very profitable to teach grammar badly'.

Even if it were accepted that research had demonstrated the uselessness of teaching *any* kind of grammar (in the narrow sense of grammatical categories and syntactic structures), it has not disposed of systematic language study (in the broader sense). Getting rid of the bathwater of grammar does not empty the bath. Watson (1987, p. 83) agrees that 'there is overwhelming evidence of the lack of any positive connection between an explicit knowledge of grammar and ability to write'. At the same time, however, he insists on the centrality of language as a focus for 'subject English'. Though he wishes that Doughty *et al.* (1971) had been 'a little less definite about the existence of a causal relationship between awareness and competence', he commends – even to 'teachers who are not committed to the language-centred model of English' – the 'sort of conscious language study' that those authors offer. The emphasis on language awareness is repeated in Watson's sympathetic quotation from Doughty *et al.*, which 'offers a form of language study which can be valued as a rewarding end in itself, namely the development of awareness. However, a basic premise of the volume is that the development of awareness in the pupil will have a positive effect upon his [*sic!*] competence, although this effect is likely to be indirect and may not show up immediately.' In so far as the prelinguistic traditional grammar was the bathwater, we are well rid of it. But the bath remains. The Kingman and Cox reports advocate a sensible refilling of the bath with systematic well-informed language study.

2 Language awareness

> Every language is a special way of looking at the world and
> interpreting experience . . . One sees and hears what the
> grammatical system of one's language has made one sensitive to, has
> trained one to look for in experience.
>
> (Clyde Kluckhohn)

What is language awareness?

Among the various speculations that looked ahead in some trepidation to the publication of the Kingman Report was the view that 'Grammar will be reinstated by Kingman, but in the form of language awareness' (National Association for the Teaching of English (NATE) Conference 1988, Newsletter). The teacher of English who said this was very probably expressing the fear that traditional prescriptive grammar (from parts of speech to figures of speech) would be restored by the Kingman Inquiry under the guise of language awareness (LA) – echoing Milton's powerful warning in *Areopagitica* that 'New Presbyter is but old Priest writ large'. But grammar has many diverse meanings. Quirk (1969, pp. 116–23) distinguished at least seven meanings. Others have since made fewer distinctions. Francis (1973, p. 137), for instance, applied to modern language a distinction between 'Grammar 1, a form of behavior; Grammar 2, a field of study; and Grammar 3, a branch of etiquette'.

Now that linguistics has become an autonomous academic subject that includes grammar (Francis's Grammar 2) as a subdivision, it is difficult for us to remember that the Greek origins of the study of grammar did not differentiate it from philosophy and logic. Grammar emerged as literally 'the art of writing'. The use of the spoken word was assigned to rhetoric, leaving grammar to deal (especially in the schoolroom) with literacy. The material for grammatical study was restricted almost entirely to written language, the language of literature and of the learned world.

> Colloquial speech in its various forms was despised and regarded as a degradation from which grammarians must save the literary style . . . grammar was given the impossible task of ascertaining the 'real' or 'true' state of the language and fixing it, at least as far as literature was concerned, in that state. (Robins, 1951, p. 44)

These assumptions established the tradition of prescriptive grammar which was to dominate Latin and English language study until the modern distinction evolved between the prescriptive (what *ought* to be said or written) and the descriptive (what *is* in fact spoken or written).

So long as which of the various 'grammars' is made clear, discussion is reasonably possible. But too often multiple ambiguity ('multiguity', as Anthony Burgess neologistically called it) prevails and causes confusion. I. A. Richards's (1938, p. 183) remark half a century ago is still sadly to the point:

> The word ['grammar'] has been pronounced, its influence descends upon the scene, and with it a strange and deadly cramp seems to spread over the intellectual faculties, afflicting them with squint, making them unable to observe all sorts of things they are perfectly conversant with in normal life.

In these circumstances it might be better to put 'grammar' into cold storage and to use more reliable terms such as 'syntax', 'morphology', 'semantics'. Many linguists have in fact dispensed altogether with the word 'grammar'.

Defining 'grammar' at all usefully illustrates strongly the difficulty of defining anything in words. Two American scholars have reminded us that 'defining must walk between two extremes of futility; the concisely erudite and the concisely oversimplified' (Lloyd and Warfel, 1956). Don Adriano de Armado, the 'fantastical Spaniard' in *Love's Labour's Lost*, enjoined his page to 'Define, define, well-educated infant'. If that was a request for precise definition, he was overestimating the possibilities of education. The most that can reasonably be demanded is an *ad hoc* definition.

The semi-technical term 'language awareness' seems to have achieved more clarification in actual use than attends the word 'grammar'. It has occurred conspicuously in educational writing in the past generation or so. Douglas Barnes's contribution to *Language, the learner and the school* (1969) ends with a few paragraphs subtitled 'Teachers' awareness of language'. He urges that 'teachers should be more *aware* of their own assumptions so that they may make explicit to pupils the criteria by which their performance will be accepted or rejected' (Barnes *et al.*, 1969, p. 35; emphasis added). In the third edition of this influential book (Barnes *et al.*, 1986, p. 30), he claims that the evidence he had collected from classrooms provided

> a basis for arguing (a) that some teachers fail to perceive the pedagogical implications of many of their own uses of language, and (b) that a descriptive study such as this provides a potential method of helping teachers to become more *aware*.

In 1975, a Schools Council Research Study recorded that 'Recent studies of reading have stressed "linguistic awareness" as something essential to reading and extra to competence in speech'. It added that 'there is clearly an area of common interest here that we need to pursue' (Britton *et al.*, 1975, p. 200).

Two articles reprinted in Mercer's *Language and Literacy* (1988) show how the same terminology has been used in the United States. G. A. Miller, reflecting on a conference on 'Language by Ear and by Eye', reported in 1972 that 'the question of *linguistic awareness* has been a central theme of this conference'

(Mercer, 1988, vol. 1, p. 215). A few years later, D. R. Olson – in a paper entitled ' "See! Jumping!" Some Oral Language Antecedents of Literacy' – argued that 'an *awareness of language* may be characterized either as a prerequisite – that is, a predisposition – to literacy or as a consequence of learning to read and write'. In his view the dilemma posed by this question had formed 'the basis of numerous studies on what is referred to somewhat infelicitously as *metalinguistic awareness*' (Mercer, ibid., p. 223).

In Britain at around the same time, Eric Hawkins produced his *Awareness of Language* (1984). He welcomed the 'explosive growth of interest in "awareness of language" as a key element in the school curriculum.' The associated Topic Books and cassette and, most of all, the forming of a Language Awareness Working Party (LAWP) focused on school-based language activities. The LAWP was sponsored by the National Congress on Languages in Education (NCLE) founded by the Centre for Information on Language Teaching and Research (CILT) which until recently occupied offices in the Carlton House headquarters of the British Council. This Council brings together foreign-language teaching of all sorts, abroad and in the United Kingdom (EFL), with English as a second language (ESL). The great majority of the language or language-related associations that have become constituent members of NCLE represent foreign-language interests. The two native-English organizations represented – NAAE (National Association of Advisers in English) and NATE (teachers) – are larger than most other bodies, but, regrettably, are as yet less committed to LA of the kind fostered by NCLE.

Strevens (1986, p. 8) has traced 'the real beginnings of language awareness' from the works of Sweet, Jespersen, H. E. Palmer and P. E. Gurrey. The University of Lancaster's Language-Ideology-Power Group argues that

> critical awareness of the world ought to be the main objective of all education, including language education. Language awareness programmes ought therefore to help children develop not only operational and descriptive knowledge of their world, but also a critical awareness of how these practices are shaped by, and shape, social relationships and relationships of power. (British Association of Applied Linguistics, Newsletter, Spring 1988, pp. 12–13)

One reason for reluctance to claim school time for LA recognizes the Law of the Conservation of the Curriculum postulated long ago by Eric (later Lord) James. This stipulated – reasonably enough – that no new subject should be proposed for an already overloaded school curriculum without specifying what should be displaced to make room for it. Though LA is usually advocated, not as a subject, but as a course, this smaller claim still requires an allotment of time that would presumably otherwise be available for the specific teaching of English or other languages. A recently retired senior member of HMI once responsible for the teaching of modern foreign languages has in fact described LA courses unfavourably as one of the 'panaceas currently in vogue'. To him, such courses seemed to be misconceived:

> The pursuit of language awareness should be an intrinsic part of learning English and the foreign languages, should arise from actual experience of language learning, should be at an appropriate conceptual level, and the planning associated with it should involve the cooperation of at least the English and modern languages departments. (Salter, 1987, p. 112)

The apparently safe position of English – or at least of English language – in British school programmes, enhanced by the extraordinary spread of English as an international language, has been contrasted with the threatened position of foreign languages other than French. This probably accounts in part for an organized LA movement being supported more strongly by foreign-language teachers and lecturers than by English specialists. Nevertheless, there are powerful academic, cultural, educational and commercial reasons for exponents of English language to be closely involved in multilingual operations. Otherwise we cannot but concede that 'It is no accident that British society is marked by a high degree of linguistic parochialism' (Hawkins, 1987, p. 13). We must, more ruefully, share with a character in Anthony Burgess's novel *Beard's Roman Women* (1977) the lament he makes in his first (and last) letter to his woman friend, Paola. After addressing her as 'tesore, amore', he admits that he would like to write in Italian but 'remains at the end a monoglot Englishman, unworthy to enter any comity of nations, tied to one tongue as to one cuisine and one insular complex of myths'. It is not merely that knowing and using a foreign language is an asset for travelling, for getting to know the country, the culture and the people for whom it is a first language. Goethe no doubt exaggerated, but he exaggerated a truth, when he wrote: 'Wer kennt nicht eine fremde Sprache, kennt nicht seine eigene' (He who doesn't know a foreign language, does not know his own). Whorf (1956, p. 244) wisely observed that 'We handle even our plain English with much greater effect if we direct it from the vantage point of a multilingual awareness'. A gloss on this, offered by Stewart Mayper, the editor of the *General Semantics Bulletin*, warned the American businessman who could see no practical value in learning foreign languages that, 'since the owners of many American businesses will be Arabs or Japanese, a "multilingual awareness" may become economically vital; he may need to understand what the English spoken by those foreigners means to *them*' (Mayper, 1986–7).

Even if it is recognized that etymological information can mislead as well as inform, familiarity with Greek and Latin terms from which English forms derive without serious change of meaning can enrich command of the lexis of English. Again, though the relevance of Greek and Latin grammatical structures has been grossly overestimated in the traditional Latinate grammar long imposed upon English, these classical languages can help to illuminate English structures by contrast if not by similarity. The comparatively slight part played by word order in Latin, for instance, emphasizes by its difference from English the sizeable role of word order rather than inflections in our language.

Against the British 'insular complex of myths' deplored by Burgess, LA (as in NCLE's LAWP) is potentially a strong weapon. In that it is a grass-roots movement, it operates, as it were, by undermining the enemy 'from the bottom upwards'. Classrooms occupying the 'bottom' level are staffed by teachers of English and foreign languages. In these circumstances, the diverse activities in them are inevitably something of a miscellany. John Sinclair, a professor of English collaborating (as the second Chairman of LAWP) with teachers of foreign languages, has described LA courses as marked, as we have noted, by 'creative untidiness'. In his *Language Awareness in Six Easy Lessons* (Sinclair 1985, pp. 33–6) he welcomes the spread by LA across the large language domain in the curriculum but tries 'to add a little stiffness to a fluid situation'. This implies an approach 'from the top down' (no invidious connotation intended!) and involves linguistic considerations – not such theoretical and exotic issues as 'umlaut in Urdu' and the like, but what is increasingly accepted as 'educational linguistics'. Broadly speaking, it is appropriate to identify a kind of hierarchy of levels. The rungs of this ladder extend from an understanding of what language *is* as an abstract universal phenomenon of human behaviour, through features of how, for what purposes and with what effectiveness languages *act* as more or less distinguishable entities, to the achievement of reasonable competence in one or more specific languages. LA explores in particular the middle ground where theorizing about language meets the practical uses of language, where de Saussure's *langue* meets his *parole*, where universals diversify into thousands of different languages.

To write, talk or even think about universal features of language necessitates using a metalanguage taken from a particular language. (It is convenient to use the term 'metalanguage' in spite of Peter Griffith's (1987, p. 43) assertion that 'There is no such thing as a metalanguage in which to talk about language, there is only language talking about language talking about language'.) In so far as language in its most general sense is a philosophical and speculative matter concerned with language-thought relationships, assumptions of universality presented less of a problem to ancient Greek and Roman philosophers (who showed little interest in other languages) than it became later in a geographically and linguistically more extensive area than the Mediterranean zone. The ancient classical languages, deemed near-perfect as instruments of thought and near-universal in validity, were assumed unquestionably to equate verbal categories with the categories of logic. Philosophical concepts such as subjects and predicates, substances and 'accidents', did not differentiate – as they needed later to do – extra-linguistic ideas from linguistic features of grammar. As the assumptions inherent particularly in Latin were transferred more or less uncritically to English, 'Distinctions were made and insisted on which were due to *a priori* speculative notions and ignored actual usage, whereas linguistic phenomena were completely ignored' (Bosker, 1947, p. 29).

The belief that the fundamental principles of grammar were the same in all languages, that is, were universal, has persisted down to modern times. When the study of historical linguistics pushed the boundaries beyond Europe and into the Far East, a Jesuit scholar, Gaston Coeurdoux, commented (in 1767) on the similarity between Sanskrit, Latin and Greek and inferred that only a common ancestor could explain it. Then the orientalist Sir William Jones in 1786 gave his famous lecture to the Bengal Asiatic Society on linguistic links establishing a common origin for all Indo-European or Aryan languages. Speculation about the origin of language came to be deplored as time-wasting. At the beginning of the twentieth century, the Linguistic Society of Paris excluded from its proceedings any papers on the subject because discussion of the topic would (in a modern linguist's words) be 'inherently unscientific and crackpot'. Nevertheless the mystery of the creation of language, without being really relevant to education or to synchronic linguistics, retains its fascination. Very recently, for example, Colin Renfrew (1987) has proposed a new location in Turkey's Anatolia as the place where human language started.

There are, of course, many non-Aryan languages, both European (for example, Finnish, Hungarian, Basque) and 'exotic'. Such was the strength of inherited beliefs, however, that nineteenth-century missionaries with amateur linguistic enthusiasm notoriously identified in the so-called 'primitive' African and Asian tongues they encountered the traditional categories (such as eight or nine parts of speech) that they had learnt to find in classical languages and consequently – if less rationally – in their own. It has remained for twentieth-century professional investigators of 'exotic' languages, notably Americans analysing Amerindian languages, to cast doubts on whether the established notions and metalinguistic terms can reasonably be perpetuated in modern languages.

Language features

By defining the subject of inquiry as 'a person's sensitivity to and conscious awareness of the nature of language and its role in human life' (Sinclair, 1985, p. 7), LA has opened up, if not 'a can of worms', at least the whole vast area covered by language and languages. John Sinclair, seeking a theoretically sound basis for an LA agenda, consulted several important works. Richard Hudson (1982) has listed 'Some Issues over which Linguists Can Agree'. His eighty or so items are grouped in three sections headed:

1 The linguistic approach to the study of language – including metalanguage as an essential tool for understanding the nature of language and of particular languages.
2 Language, society and the individual – including linguistic universals; dialects; English as a world language; varieties of language; Standard English; Received Pronunciation; change; acquisition; speech as behaviour.
3 The structure of language – including pronunciation; writing; spelling; vocabulary; syntax; meaning.

Doing justice even to most of these issues, however, would need far more time than is, or is likely to become, available in schools.

The American C. F. Hockett (from another of whose works we have already quoted – see page 11) wrote in 1961 a paper on 'The Problem of Universals in Language' reprinted in Hockett 1977. A language universal, he said, is 'a feature or property shared by all language'. Hockett compared human language with animal communication systems in order to list grammatical universals. Here again, the number of generalizations (nearly fifty) which he found is still too great for schools to cope with. John Lyons selected from Hockett's list four 'key' language features, calling them

1 Arbitrariness – lack of the iconicity which makes forms actually resemble meanings.
2 Duality – two levels of structure, phonological and grammatical.
3 Productivity – Hockett's *openness*, the property enabling users to coin innumerable new utterances not previously encountered.
4 Discreteness – word-forms being either absolutely the same or absolutely different (unlike the signal-elements in, say, bee-dancing, where they can be 'graded' according to intensity or orientation).

Sinclair commends this specification, especially for comparing and contrasting human verbal communication with the systems used by bees and mammalians (such as apes, dolphins). Nevertheless, he finds the Lyons' categories rather abstract for the purpose of teaching average pupils. He accordingly modifies them, producing his *Six Easy Lessons* (1985). The 'central and crucial features of language' which he finds most appropriate to the practical needs of classes are:

1 Productivity – as characterized by Lyons.
2 Creativity – including the breaking of conventional rules, poetic licence and use of metaphor, and presumably including features of what Hockett calls *prevarication*, whereby messages can be false, obscure or meaningless.
3 Stability and change – contrasting relative fixedness with long-term fluidity and daily neologism.
4 Social variation – variety of languages, and associated paralinguistic and extra-linguistic features.
5 How to do things with language – individual variation leading to variable interpretation.
6 The two-layered code – corresponding to the *interchangeability* named by Hockett and Lyons, indicating features whereby individuals in conversation or discourse alternate between sending and receiving messages.

The various specifications mentioned above reflect the interweaving of the features characterizing the whole complex of language. Whichever path one takes for entry into the maze, it is likely to diverge in many directions, offering various routes for exploring the whole territory. For example, a narrow path representing a specific form of punctuation such as *hyphenation* might lead to the concept of a *word*, raising problems of definition (is a hyphened item such as 'flower-pot' one word, the same as 'flowerpot', or two words like 'flower pot'?), of differentiation (does speech use words equivalent to those visually presented in writing? in what respects is rhetorical punctuation different from grammatical punctuation?). More generally, is punctuation necessary? Are there other features of punctuation (for example, the possessive apostrophe) which are more or less dispensable and at what cost? How does English punctuation differ from other systems (cf. the Spanish use of question marks in '¿Quién es ese caballero?')? And so on.

Alternatively, venturing on a semantic path, consider *jargon*. Does this confront the explorer with choices (linguistically because of polysemy) leading perhaps to (a) the Old French *jargonner* equivalent to the warbling, twittering or chattering of birds comparable with the 'sweet *jargonning*' of the birds in *The Rime of the Ancient Mariner* or to (b) the modern child's 'scribble-talk' (Crystal's label, 1987a, p. 35) or to (c) the 'insider' language used satisfactorily within a group of specialists but displayed objectionably, often unintelligibly, to 'outsiders', or to (d) the gobbledegook of -ese language (officialese, legalese, journalese, sociologese, motherese, educationalists' pedagoguese) or of American 'globaloney' and 'psychobabble'? The last of these produces the 'sybaritic miasma' in which, for instance, separated marital partners in Cyra McFadden's *The Serial* have 'a good rap about redefining the parameters of our interface'. These considerations converge on the capacity of language to generate ambiguity, ranging from the essentially literary ambiguity of Empson's *Seven Types* to the disreputable deceptions of doublespeak, of a language 'full of sound and fury dignifying nothing' and responsible – again in Thurber's words – for 'the havoc wrought by verbal artillery on the fortress of reason'.

3 The semantic dimension

'Meaning' is a harlot among words; it is a temptress who can seduce the writer or speaker from the paths of intellectual chastity.

(Colin Cherry)

Forms and meanings

All verbal languages are uttered through forms, phonic or graphic. But linguistic forms are used primarily to express, to grasp, to communicate meanings. Anthony Burgess, reviewing in the *Observer*, 20 July 1986, a scholarly book on *The Origin of Writing* (Harris, 1986), remarked significantly: 'The alphabet may be exalted by linguists, who hear speech as the primal reality, but the linguists are being overtaken by the semiologists whose epoch this is.' This ought to be good news for teachers, whose main job after all is to teach sets of meanings called 'subjects'. But many, perhaps most, teachers of mother-tongue English seem to remain suspicious and fearful of what they apprehend as 'linguistics', which nowadays can include 'semantics'. Teachers of English as a second or foreign language are probably less antipathetic. So, apparently, are continental Europeans. In a Unesco monograph prepared for the International Bureau of Education, the writer (using English) remarks: 'We feel . . . that an initiation to the complexity of the phenomena of meaning is indispensable to the training of all primary- and secondary-level teachers' (Bronckart, 1985, p. 59).

The fairly popular term 'semantics' is applied to the whole territory of meaning, but more technically it has been restricted to semiology or semiotics – the study of the theory of signs, particularly word-signs. Morris (1946, p. 222) divides semiotics into three parts, of which semantics is only one. His three interdependent areas are designated:

1 Syntactics – signs and the relations between signs.
2 Semantics – signs and the experiences (real or imagined) they designate, that is, the *designata*.
3 Pragmatics – signs and their relations to users.

Language teachers, employed to help learners to *use* languages, are naturally most interested in pragmatics, but of the three semiotic areas this has been the most neglected. One reason for this is the sheer complexity and elusive character of anything to do with meaning. One linguist adjures us to 'pity the poor analyst, who has to do the best he can with meanings that are as elusive as a piece of soap in a bathtub' (Bolinger, 1975, p. 205). A critic went further with lines satirizing semantics in the broadest sense:

> Semantics will make it clear to you
> That black is white –
> When looked at from the proper point of view.
> And eminent semanticists will undertake to show
> That Yes is but a neater form of No.
>   (Ruby, 1956)

A more serious reason for the neglect turns on the relationship between teachers and linguists (or rather, linguisticians – experts in the study of language). The twentieth century has seen an 'explosion' in linguistic studies. It might therefore seem natural and reasonable for language teachers to seek guidance from the increasing number of reputable students of language. As early as 1903, Victoria Welby noted that 'some of the most distinguished experts in language – notably Michel Bréal and Dr Postgate – have begun to protest in plain terms against the prevailing neglect by linguistic scholars of Semantics, the science of the change of meaning.' But her hopes of a renewed interest in the semantic dimension were not fulfilled. For much of the century, linguistics was dominated by the 'excluded meaning' principle favoured by supporters of the theories of behaviourist psychology. In his influential *Language*, the American Leonard Bloomfield abandoned his earlier 'mentalist' position and defined the meaning of linguistic forms in behaviourist stimulus-response terms. He rated the statement of meanings as 'the weak-point in language study', excluded it from the territory of linguistics and expected it to 'remain so until human knowledge advances very far beyond its present state' (Bloomfield, 1933, p. 140). Consequently he has been thought responsible for the 'virtual death-knell of semantics in the U.S.A. for the next twenty years' (Leech, 1974, p. 3).

Being vigorous advocates of 'structuralism', the Americans Bloch and Trager in 1942 based their *Outline of Linguistic Analysis* on the theory that all their 'classifications must be based exclusively on FORM' and that 'there must be no appeal to meaning, to abstract logic, or to philosophy'. Even if their work had been successful in producing a description of language totally divorced from semantics, it would have been of little use to language teachers and other educationists, for whom language exists primarily to negotiate meanings. It would, in the terms of another linguist, have succeeded only in 'setting up a code book without a key'. Some years after the publication of the *Outline*, Bloch himself conceded that 'meaning, at least, is so obviously useful as a short cut in the investigation of phonemic structure . . . that any linguist who refused to employ it would be very largely wasting his time'.

The 'behaviourist period' dominated the linguistic scene until Chomsky's famous assault in 1959 on B. F. Skinner's *Verbal Behavior* (1957). In England, at much the same time, Quirk (1960, p. 57) detected 'signs that even those American groups who have followed a different course in the name of Bloomfield are now realizing that only relatively coarse-meshed statements can be made if the consideration of meaning is rigorously excluded'. The 'reinstatement of meaning as a legitimate and fruitful topic of general linguistic enquiry' was also recognized by Harris (1987, p. 89). Meanwhile semantics has served Ogden and Richards (1923) (see p. 89) and the semantic differential devised by Osgood and his colleagues. Of more specifically grammatical relevance has been the development in Britain of systemic grammar. Butler (1985) refers variously to 'semantic functional grammar', 'semantically significant grammar', 'semanticized grammar' and 'semantically oriented grammar'. Michael Halliday, closely associated from the first with systemic analysis, has produced, also in 1985, *An Introduction to Functional Grammar* based on systemic theory. In it he seeks to account for how language is *used*, and examines 'how and why an individual makes choices from the syntactic structures and vocabulary available, according to the meaning being conveyed'.

Language teachers who free themselves from the assumptions embedded in a subject-based school curriculum are faced with a sizeable number of challenges. These are presented in:

(a) the recommendations of the Kingman Report (DES, 1988) on the study of the English language;
(b) the recommendations of the Bullock Report (DES, 1975), especially favouring language across the curriculum;
(c) the recognition of the centrality of meaning in that, in Dewey's words, language is for 'organizing our thoughts about things';
(d) the advocacy of an awareness of the phenomenon of language in general and of a range of languages relevant to educational contexts.

Language-awareness activities focus particularly on the last two of these.

To some extent, using words can be seen as an obverse of watching 'movies'. Whereas film projects a series of still photographs to create the illusion of continuous movement, language cuts up the continuous flowing of human experience into momentarily static segments. In more abstract terms, it interrupts the continuum of meaning by classifying mental concepts into word categories. Intelligence, it has been said, 'breaks up the fluid continuity of the Universe into sharply definite, easily manageable, conceptualized entities.' In doing so, 'it falsifies the true nature of Reality' (Passmore, 1970, pp. 242–3). Consequently, the world objectified by language cannot completely or with total accuracy reflect the essential 'true' reality of existence. (Mystical intuitions may conceivably, as Bergson and others believed, get nearer to absolute truth – if it exists – but intuition is an extra-linguistic phenomenon.) It follows that language cannot but be approximate, using categories and distinctions that are themselves relatively approximate, indeterminate and 'fuzzy' – with fuzzy demarcations, edges, borders, boundaries, ambiguities, deceptions and vaguenesses.

Language grids

Being approximate in character, language manages to achieve more or less, but rarely perfect, 'closeness of verbal fit'. Different languages, of course, vary in the degree of 'closeness' they achieve. They map meanings – more of less equivalent meanings, as far as we can comprehend the cognitive processes involved – in more or less different ways. In a popular linguistic metaphor, they use different 'grids' for fitting words to meanings. Echoing the phrases of Whorf when expounding the famous Whorf–Sapir hypothesis, Catford (1959, p. 182) argues that our language 'provides a kind of grid, or series of grids, through which we "see" the world, dissected along lines laid down by the systems of the language'.

The most thoroughly explored 'grids' are those investigating the semantic fields of the terminology of colour. Here the standard work (Berlin and Kay, 1969) analyses colour vocabulary in eighty or so languages. It is not surprising that all languages reflect perceptions of colour (no language has only one colour term!) and all have terms for black and white. Given the enormously varying sizes of dictionaries, demonstrated by the weights of different monolingual dictionaries, it is obvious that some languages make more distinctions than others: English relies on 11 basic colour words, while many others seem to manage with fewer. According to Brunelle (1973), Whorf for instance found that the language of Hopi Indians did not distinguish blue from green. More interestingly, boundaries are placed differently. Martinet (1960, p. 21) equates the French 'blue' and 'green' zones with Welsh and Breton '*glas*', but Robins (1964, p. 72) complicates things by equating Welsh '*glas*' with English 'green', 'blue' and 'grey' and by adding that the colour brown was shared among Welsh 'glas',

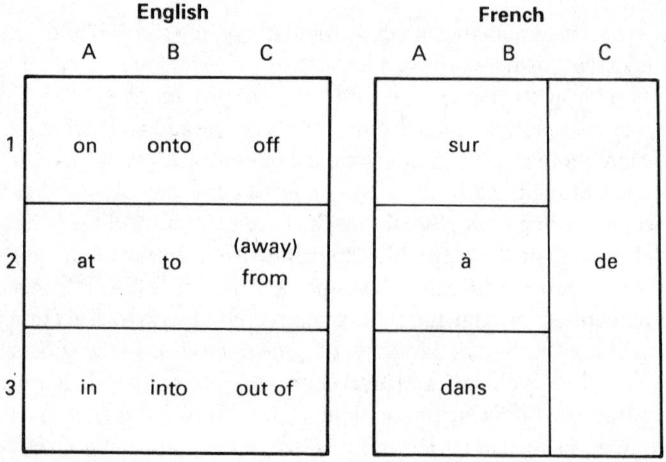

Figure 1   Prepositions
Derived from Catford (1959, pp. 184–5)

'gwrydd' and 'llwyd'. Clearly colour perceptions do not precisely match colour terminologies.

The English language, compared with many others, seems to overwork the verb 'to know' by applying it to both abstract and concrete experiences, making it cover 'knowing that' as well as 'knowing how', that is, 'being familiar with a fact' as well as 'being acquainted with someone'. Both Romance and Germanic languages commonly use two words to make such differentiations – e.g. German 'wissen'/'kennen', Dutch 'weten'/'kennen', French 'savoir'/'connaître', Spanish 'saber'/'conocer', Russian 'znat''/'umet''.

A simple example comparing the preposition systems of two familiar languages – English and French – was used by Catford (1959, pp. 184–5) in a lecture on 'English as a Foreign Language'. This showed the contrast in two parallel charts (Figure 1). As the diagrammatic arrangement shows, columns indicate respectively differentiation between words denoting spatial relations of (A) static contiguity, (B) dynamic approach or arrival, and (C) dynamic departure or separation; the rows represent end-point positions that are (1) exterior, (2) indifferently exterior or interior, and (3) interior. The French grid conflates columns A and B and, under C, rows 1–3. The fact that French needs only four prepositions to do the work of nine English prepositions does not, of course, imply that French speakers lack cognitive semantic distinctions that are separately expressed in single English words. If English, as we are assured, has a vocabulary at least twice as large as those of French, German, Spanish and Italian, it presumably makes a much larger number of simple *verbal* distinctions. But, contrary to C. S. Lewis's assertion (1967, p. 6) that 'The language which can with the greatest ease make the finest and most numerous distinctions of meaning is the best', there is no virtue in multiplying distinctions beyond necessity.

An obvious tit-for-tat argument with which to counter the simplistic case for rating English above French in 'number-crunching' terms would be that French uses three words for the concept of time where English relies on a single one. A rival chart might be set up as follows:

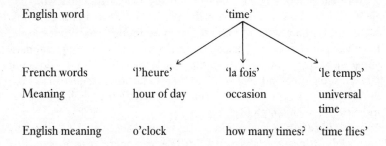

English word		'time'	
French words	'l'heure'	'la fois'	'le temps'
Meaning	hour of day	occasion	universal time
English meaning	o'clock	how many times?	'time flies'

French 'temps' also embraces English 'weather', adding further complications to English–French correspondences.

A similar example taken from German presents a battery of words equivalent to the English 'before':

		German
1 Spatially in front of (He stood *before* the mirror)	corresponding to	'vor'
2 Temporally in advance of (I'll see you *before* you leave)		'ehe', 'bevor'
3 Formerly in time (I've read this *before*)		vorher, im voraus

On the other hand German 'stoßen' seems to represent various kinds of hitting, meaning in English:

'kick' – strike with the foot
'nudge' – push with the elbow
'prod' – poke with a pointed stick.

Even more semantically elusive are the various differentiations categorized variously by these two languages. Thus, the field of knowledge and understanding is divided up by three lexemes in Middle High German. These, John Lyons (1981b) tells us, correspond more or less to Platonic Greek's 'technē', 'epistēmē' and 'sophiā' and are translatable into English by the words 'art', 'knowledge' (or 'science') and 'wisdom'.

Such asymmetric correspondences sometimes appear to be caused by the sheer arbitrariness of language. At other times there may be an influence of cultural differences. Eskimos are often mentioned as having no single general-purpose term for snow but a range of words according to variation of condition and usefulness (hard-packed and therefore suitable for igloo-building, or crisp, or slushy). Obviously this circumstance is culture-specific. Less well-known is the apparent fact that Argentinian gauchos use only a few plant names but have very many expressions denoting the colours of horses' hides – though it would be remarkable if the latter class includes as many as the alleged two hundred terms. Presumably it is the importance of bullfighting in Spain that contributes to the Spanish language a specific term ('patas') for the legs of bulls and other animals, distinguishing them from human legs ('piernas'). Russian – it is said – does not differentiate between 'foot' and 'leg' after the English fashion, but distributes the relevant limblike meanings among a furniture leg ('nóska'), the whole animal leg ('nóga') and a twelve-inch length ('fut').

A further complication, even within a single language, can be caused by innovations which dislocate established grids. Before credit cards were introduced, 'pay by cash or cheque' meant 'use currency (cash, banknotes) or cheques'. The new development produced 'pay by cash or credit card', stretching 'cash' to include cheques as well as cash, jointly opposed to plastic cards.

Metaphors and hedges

Even if these equivalences are reported only with partial reliability, they tempt us to contemplate awareness of metaphor, a fascinating but bewildering phenomenon. Wittgenstein acknowledged its significance with his image of metaphor as a net thrown over reality. A furniture 'leg' is clearly and trivially metaphorical – a 'dead' metaphor. But it is possible to see 'live' metaphor, as do Lakoff and Johnson (1980), as central to language and hence to our conceptual system and to our whole *Weltanschauung*. So large and strong is the temptation to explore the universe of metaphor that it must, in the interests of time and space, be resisted. (We shall, however, glance at it again in Chapter 5.)

The relevance of variable language grids is, as we have noted, also of prime importance to translation. The meanings conveyed by words exist mysteriously and unreachably between the ears. When 'retrieved' as much as is feasible, they probably never match with exactitude their denotations – let alone their connotations. Whether we like it or not, users of all languages need to enter into what has been called 'a contract of incertitude', relying – among other things – on 'hedging' systems (see Skelton, 1988, pp. 37, 39). Academic language notoriously favours caution, though the report of a conversation between two professors walking in the countryside –

'The sheep seem to have been shorn.'
'Apparently so, on *this* side.'

– is probably fictitious and certainly exaggerated. Popular English 'hedges' – sometimes protecting the subtext implicit in 'coded language' – include modifying items such as 'so to speak', 'as it were', 'strictly speaking', 'technically', 'a veritable', as well as verbs such as 'seem', 'appear', modal verb forms, adverbs like 'quite', 'rather', 'often', and so on. Lakoff (1975, p. 221) claims that

students of language, especially psychologists and linguistic philosophers, have long been attuned to the fact that natural language concepts have vague boundaries and fuzzy edges and that, consequently, natural language sentences will often be neither true, nor false, nor nonsensical, but rather true to a certain extent and false to a certain extent, true in certain respects and false in other respects.

Failure to accept 'hedges' can lead to the kind of plight which Simone de Beauvoir (1958, p. 26) reports in her autobiographical writings. She confesses to having had instilled into her by adults the assumption that language – presumably not just her own French language – fits reality exactly:

Puisque j'échouais à penser sans le secours du langage, je supposais que celui-ci couvrait exactement la réalité; j'y étais initiée par les adultes que je prenais pour les dépositaires de l'absolu: en designant une chose, ils en exprimaient la substance, au sens où l'on exprime le jus d'un fruit.

James Kirkup (de Beauvoir, *Memoirs*, Bk I, 1959, p. xxx) translates this as follows:

Since I failed to think without the help of language, I supposed that the latter exactly represented reality; I was initiated into that belief by the adults whom I took as the repositories of the absolute: in indicating a thing they exposed its substance, just as one presses out the juice of a fruit.

She went on to describe how the collapse of this induced assumption caused her sense of truth to fade away:

The world around me was harmoniously based on fixed coordinates [*coordonnées fixes*] and divided into clear-cut compartments [*catégories tranchées*]. No neutral tints were allowed: everything was in black and white; there was no intermediate position between the traitor and the hero, the renegade and the martyr; all inedible fruits were poisonous; I was told I 'loved' every member of my family, including my most ill-favoured great-aunts. All my experience belied this essentialism. White was only rarely totally white, and the blackness of evil was relieved by lighter touches; I saw greys and half-tones everywhere. Only as soon as I tried to define their muted shades, I had to use words, and I found myself in a world of bony-structured concepts. Whatever I beheld with my own eyes and every real experience had to be fitted somehow or other into a rigid category; the myths and the stereotyped ideas prevailed over the truth: unable to pin it down, I allowed truth to dwindle into insignificance.

The passage quoted above in French reveals several features of quasi-equivalence between the two languages. It ends with a sentence using 'exprimer' twice – 'ils en *exprimaient* la substance, au sens où l'on *exprime* le jus d'un fruit'. This might conceivably be a clever play – almost a pun – on the verb. In any case, it exploits two rather different but distantly related meanings. A standard French-English dictionary (Harrap's) equates 'exprimer' with two English phrases – 'to put into words' and 'to squeeze out'. The citation supporting the second meaning – 'exprimer le jus d'un citron' – is coincidentally almost identical with de Beauvoir's final words. An etymological dictionary of the English language interestingly traces our 'express' back through Middle English 'espressen' and Old French 'espresser, expresser' to a combination of Latin 'ex' and 'pressare', the latter being a frequentative verb derived from 'premere' (to press). The sense of physically pressing survives in modern English 'cider-press' and keep-fit 'press-ups', but more commonly serves the fourth estate, the printing Press.

School learners of French (alongside English), if emancipated from the myth of single exact word-meanings, should appreciate – and might be fascinated by – the semi-equivalences demonstrated by the two language grids. Translation problems might start with simple terms such as 'bonjour' (more or less 'good day'), 'cul-de-sac', 'enfant terrible', 'bagatelle', 'entre nous' (less rather than more equivalent to 'between us'), 'faux pas' (figurative 'false step' but more exactly a 'social blunder'), 'faute de mieux' (neater than the stilted 'for lack of anything better'), 'nouveau riche' (vulgarly new-rich), 'cause célèbre' (famous law-suit or controversy), 'femme fatale' (seductive woman). These French items, with definitions, are actually recorded in some monolingual *English* dictionaries.

So is 'sang-froid' (composure, calmness), but of course without the familiar mistranslation of 'l'Anglais avec son sang-froid habituel' into 'the Englishman with his usual bloody cold'. More metaphorical loans might include 'ballon d'essai' (figuratively, kite-flying) and the untranslatable 'esprit d'escalier'. Our tabloid Press has recently made an addition to the list with 'un lapin chaud', a 'hot rabbit' being the picturesque phrase for a woman-chaser. The victim of this locution was the current French President.

Our own Prime Minister (notre Dame de Fer) was recently said to have used her visit to Bruges and her attack on the notion of united nations of Europe as an opportunity 'pour épater les bourgeois'. The difficulty of adequately translating 'bourgeois', and therefore the whole phrase containing it, raises questions about the status of this and many other loan-words. A 'loan scale' for words borrowed by English from French would stretch from those (such as souvenir, coup, genre, voyeur) so completely Anglicized as to lose their distinctive semantic Frenchness to others less completely assimilated (such as 'droit de seigneur', 'pis aller', 'de trop'). Along with the latter would probably belong those which in print, even if not regularly italicized, usually retain – at least in lower case – French accents (as in 'idée fixe', 'déjà vu', 'à la carte', 'bête noire', 'pièce de résistance'). A marginal case would be 'façade', often shedding the cedilla in its Anglicized form.

Faux amis

A related phenomenon often affecting translation or mistranslation is that of *faux amis* (sometimes rendered in English somewhat over-literally as 'false friends'). The French phrase was coined by M. Koessler and J. Derocquigny in *Les Faux-amis ou les trahisons du vocabulaire anglais; conseils aux traducteurs* (1928). The apparent frequency of 'false' Anglo-French friendships has been explored in a whole book by Thody and Evans (1985). Their title – *Faux amis and key words* – emphasizes the cultural and social roots of vocabularies. The 'lookalikes and confusables' phrase implies that English learners of French – for instance, in educational institutions – can be confused by graphic similarities seeming falsely to indicate identity of meaning. First encounters with the French language inevitably produce confusion between forms such as 'parents', meaning 'father and mother' in English but, more extensively, 'relatives' in French. The catalogue of *faux amis* can be divided very roughly into sets according to how 'confusability' can range from the very unlikely to the only too possible. These are more or less ordered from less to more likely in a short sample:

French		*English*
le pain	(not pain, but)	bread
les boucles	(not buckles, but)	curls
l'essence	(not essence, but)	petrol
le couvert	(not cover, but)	knife, fork and spoon
la garniture (de frein)	(not garniture, but)	brake-lining

French		*English*
actuel	(not actual, but)	real, present (in time)
la réclamation	(not reclamation, but)	complaint
le transatlantique	(not transatlantic, but)	deck-chair
verifier	(not verify, but)	check
les prunes	(not prunes, but)	plums
un contrôleur	(not a controller, but)	a guard.

Wallace Chafe (1968, p. 602) was surely not thinking solely of English when he described language as 'a remarkably complicated elephant'. All languages are complicated; even more so are the relationships between or among them. Writing under the title 'Parlez-vous Business?', about Franglais, frenchifying and francization, Chris Leeds (1988, No. 3) illustrates the to-and-fro oscillation between English and French with, appropriately enough, the word 'tennis'. Apparently this word originally Anglicized French 'tenez' but it has returned to modern French as 'tennis'. Similarly, the now obsolete 'la bougette' (purse, pouch) was borrowed in the seventeenth century for English 'budget', only for that form to be exported back to France as 'le budget'. The falsely friendly mistake whereby 'l'occasion' is sometimes mistranslated as English 'occasion' instead of 'opportunity' or 'bargain' has recoiled through a frenchified use of 'opportunité'. One cannot imagine the French Academy tolerating such an invasion, but it must find it harder to resist the adoption of the neatly simple 'jet-lag' in place of the 'pure' but cumbersome French 'décalage horaire'.

In principle, any pair of languages in close contact can generate the equivalent of Franglais ('Japlish' and 'Itangliano' – Japanese/English and Italian/English – are recent recruits) and, inevitably, *faux amis*. The growing popularity and alleged success of dual-language texts for collaborative reading in multicultural British schools has already produced books and 'support packs' twinning English with Bengali, Punjabi and Gujarati; it would be strange if this development did not throw up some *faux amis*. The existence of such things between European languages has long been recognized. For German, the deceptive 'bekommen' is well known from the anecdote about the German who, having waited impatiently for his café breakfast, plaintively asked: 'When do I become a sausage?' Other mistranslations, probably less apocryphal, turn on:

German		*English*
Fleisch	(not flesh, but)	meat
Schwein	(not swine, but)	pork
Rechnung	(not reckoning, but)	bill
Brief	(not brief, but)	letter
Prüfen	(not prove, but)	test

Identical spellings in two languages emphasize how likely or unlikely are assumptions of identical meanings. 'Brief' is protected from ambiguity by wide difference between the German noun meaning 'a letter' and the English adjective meaning 'short'. On the other hand, the title '*Also* sprach Zarathrustra' could easily be mistranslated into 'Z *also* spoke' instead of, correctly, 'Z spoke *thus*'.

Anglo-Italian items of the same kind include:

Italian		*English*
camera	(not camera, but)	room
colazione	(not collation, but)	breakfast
caldo	(not cold, but)	warm
pantalone	(not pantaloons, but)	trousers

Such is the foreignness of Old English, despite its continuity with modern English, that an American book (Barney, 1977) offers to students warnings against confusing vocabulary items:

Anglo-Saxon	*Modern English*	
cræftig	powerful	(not normally 'crafty')
dom	judgement	(not normally 'doom')
rice	powerful	(not normally 'rich')
sellan	give	(not normally 'sell')
slean	strike	(not normally 'slay')
þyncan	seem	(not normally 'think')
wiþ	against	(not normally 'with')

As 1992 approaches, development of a single European market emphasizes the multilingual importance, especially to insular Britain, of language transfer and of translation. Transfer includes the phenomena of language grids, while translation (see Chapter 10) is attended by a current revival of interest in computerized translation.

4 Conventional and deviant language

> Conventional English is the twin sister to barren thought.
> (A. N. Whitehead)

The book you are reading seeks to deal with features shared by many languages. Its purpose consequently suffers from various limitations. Its text uses basically a single language – Standard English. Being written, it necessarily employs specific graphic forms for conveying its meanings. Its writer is not in any strict sense bilingual, his monolingualism being diluted only to a slight extent by his limited acquaintance with one or two European languages. Bearing in mind these limitations, he will try to avoid excessive monoglot parochialism when considering Sinclair's (1985) six propositions about 'central and crucial features of language'. In Sinclair's terminology, these propositions are: productivity; creativity; stability and change; social variation; how to do things with language; and the two-layered code (see page 27 above). Obviously there are considerable overlaps among the six. Instead of attempting (and probably failing) to give preliminary definitions, we shall operate *solvitur ambulando*, hoping that workable distinctions will be sufficiently implied by what is included under the various headings.

Productivity and openness

This feature can be taken to fall short of being 'creative' or 'original', whatever those notoriously vague terms mean. Even so, productivity is a remarkable phenomenon, reflecting the capacity of a *finite* vocabulary, in a variety of syntactic arrangements, to generate an *infinite* number of utterances. These phonological or graphic 'strings' range from more ordinary, pedestrian, prosaic sentences that have not before been knowingly said or written to utterances which are distinctly imaginative, even poetic. An arbitrary demarcation can defer poetic uses of language for consideration under 'creativity', understood as a kind of productivity-plus.

Some linguists, such as the aforementioned Hockett, label our 'productivity' as 'openness'. This calls to mind the important distinction between '*open* classes' and '*closed* sets' of words. The former are the more productive, in the sense that class membership is infinitely extendable, whereas 'closed sets' (for example, systems of personal pronouns or prepositions) rarely accept new members. (An exception is the feminist addition of 'Ms' to the small set of terms of address.) To some extent this distinction corresponds to another one, between words that are intrinsically significant and those that are significant only by linking structurally with other words. And this is related, in technical terminology, to the old syntagmatic/paradigmatic differentiation.

The long history of this distinction can be traced as far back as to Aristotle. Later, in the sixth century AD, Priscian introduced it in Latin by distinguishing 'significantia' from 'consignificantia'. Medieval writers about language used the Greek-derived synonyms 'categoremata' and 'syncategoremata'. In some eighteenth-century English theorizing (for example, by Horne Tooke) essentially the same distinction persisted under the names of 'Principals' and 'Abbreviations'. Here the labels gave, as the pro-Latin tradition dictated, a higher status to the former (characteristically declinable) forms than to the downgraded latter (normally indeclinable) forms. A less biased naming preferred the neutral terms 'autosemantic' and 'synsemantic'. The second of these titles removed much of the stigma from Particles (mainly prepositions, conjunctions, pronouns, articles, demonstratives, interjections, and some adverbs) which otherwise were dismissed – for instance, in *A New Grammar* (1745?), attributed to Ann Fisher – as 'little odd trifling Words' lacking the prestige of proper inflected parts of speech. Presumably it was this prejudice that prolonged the practice, in many early school grammars of English, of wrongly numbering participles (which had long before shed their Old English inflexional endings) among the *declinable* parts of speech. (The Latin equivalents remain, of course, inflectable.)

Crystal (1987b, p. 407) offers a diagrammatic representation of the syntagmatic/paradigmatic differentiation:

```
                    Syntagmatic
           ───────────────────────────────────►
      P
      a    She    +   can     +   go
      r     .          .           .
      a     .          .           .
      d     .          .           .
      i    He         will        run
      g    I          may         sit
      m    You        might       see
      a
      t
      i
      c  ↓ etc.       etc.        etc.
```

Here the + symbols join the items that make up the syntax of the simple sentences (subject + modal auxiliary + lexical verb). Syntax, a comparatively stable feature of English, is more 'closed', more restricted to the ordering of closed-set components. The subject is necessarily a *noun*-like term (noun, pronoun, gerund, infinitive); the rest (traditionally called a predicate) is based on a *verb*-like term.

The horizontal 'syntagmatic' arrow indicates that syntax does extend. It does so, for instance, by adding objects, complements, adverbs, clauses, and so on. But extensions are not productive in the innovatory sense of that term. Deviant innovations within English syntax, and doubtless in other languages, are numerically rare. One example in spoken English might be, or might once have been, novel in the language used in radio broadcasts. The special circumstances of that medium, associated with special intonation patterns, allowed BBC broadcasters to say:

And so, until tomorrow, it's goodbye from us.

Northern Ireland – and the government has agreed to hold an inquiry.

Cricket – and play resumed at Headingley this morning.

Comparable syntactic innovations in print – limiting ourselves to English – might include oddities characteristic of other special language registers. One golf club professional, for example, advertised for sale his stock of footwear as

GOLF SHOES, THE STUDS WON'T WEAR OUT.

The combination of ellipsis – [Here are for sale] golf shoes, the studs [of which] won't wear out – and defiance of normal syntactic arrangements (are those 'shoes' in the nominative, accusative – or even vocative – grammatical case?) nevertheless triumphs communicatively. In a more academic context, one impressive linguistic abstracting periodical (the American *Language and Language Behavior Abstracts*) has for years used an unusual syntactic formula which reverses the normal order of 'to be' auxiliary verbs and past participles. Many of their summaries begin with sentences such as:

Examined is the psychological status of . . .

Investigated were adult and child syntactic strategies . . .

Refuted is the assumption that . . .

Listed and cross-referenced are 1,047 words . . .

Presumably such unusual syntax is at least quasi-productive in that it produces economy in newsprint.

Another deviant use of English that is productive by producing a 'new' language is so-called pidgin English. This seems to combine lexical variants which are not neologistic in form so much as semantic substitutions of standard quasi-synonyms (for example, 'coconut' for 'head') with more important innovations in syntax. The remark 'That fellow coconut belong him no grass' ('He's bald') resists conventional clause analysis. The popular 'belong' construction replacing possessive pronominals is also used in 'Belly blong me walk about too much' ('I was seasick') and in the highly inventive 'Him kerosene blong Jesus Christ bimeby all gone, bugger up, finish' (There has been an eclipse!) It has been suggested that pidgins (Dutch, French, Portuguese, etc. as well as English) adapted their home languages to match relevant foreign languages, particularly Chinese.

The putative Far East connexion is, as it were, reversed in the following (probably apocryphal) composition allegedly written by an Oriental student living in England. The syntax, unlike that of the pidgin English sentences quoted, is more or less normal, but its vocabulary, its grammatical concord and its spelling are extraordinarily deviant:

> The banana are a great remarkable fruit. He are constructed in the same architectural style as the honorable sausage. Difference being skin of sausage are habitually consumed, while it not advisable to eat rapping of banana. Perhaps also intrissing the following differences between the two objects. Banana are held aloft while consuming, sausage are usually left in reclining position. Banana are first green culler then gradual turn yellowish. Sausage start out with indifinite culler (resemble terrier cotta) and retain same hue indefinitely. Sausage depend for creation upon human being or stuffing machine, while banana are pristine product of honorable mother nature. Both article resemble the other in that neither have pit or colonel of any kind.

With relevance to a European language, one recalls a wartime issue of *Punch* which picked on the German tendency syntactically to postpone main verbs to clause-final position. Referring to a report of the abandonment of a scheme to release coalminers for military service by replacing them in the mines with young boys, it remarked facetiously:

> Boys down coal-mines will be dropped. Ja, ach!

A parody of a warning sign displayed alongside a massive early computer announced, in a mixture of German and English:

> *Achtung! Allen Lookenpeepers!*
> Das Computermaschine is nicht fur gefingerpoken und mittengraben. Is easy schaden der springenwerk, blowenfusen, und spitzensparken. Is nicht fur gewerken by das Dummkopfen . . .

Here the syntax is basically that of standard English.

Turning more specifically from the syntactic to the paradigmatic, and therefore to open-set words, we can draw again on Crystal's diagram above (page 41). In it, the vertical columns contain dots indicating 'and so on' and end with 'etc.'s. These mark the extendability of each column by possible additions of countless other subjects and verbs (for example, 'Power + tends to + corrupt').

All known languages have open classes of words; most languages have closed sets. Simple English language categories (using mainly traditional names) are:

(a) open – noun, adjective, verb
(b) closed – article, demonstrative pronoun, conjunction, preposition.

(Adverbs, belonging to a miscellaneous 'ragbag' category, cannot be clearly assigned to either type; Horne Tooke referred to them as 'the common sink and repository of all heterogeneous and unknown corruptions'.) Prepositions to a slight degree span both classes, leaving the 'closed' door ajar. A single word 'onto', long refused entry, is now accepted, and the Scottish 'outwith' has been admitted. Since 'uptil' has been seen, it may one day gain entry. Aitchison (1987, p. 104) quotes as new prepositions 'upsides', meaning 'up alongside', 'up beside', and (in the register of sailing) 'overside'. Open classes being indefinitely extendable, anyone can invent a new proper noun (for example, hypocorisms such as 'Jennykins' in baby-language or motherese, or the *Guardian*'s 'Niglet' for a previous Chancellor of the Exchequer). Lewis Carroll was particularly inventive in extending our categories of adjectives (slithy, vorpal, uffish, etc.) and verbs (galumphing, burbled, gyre, outgrabe, etc.).

Nonsense and neologism

Carroll's 'nonsense' verse is comprehensible after a fashion. Some of it has been 'acted' dramatically by primary school children and 'Jabberwocky' has been translated into French, German and other foreign languages – and must consequently to some extent have a sort of meaning. This is largely so because the orthodox functors or 'form-words', as well as significant affixes (such as pre- and -ing), are retained and maintain the structure supporting the contentives or 'content words'. Structures are therefore ordered syntactically in conventional English sentence patterns. The fact that in English syntactic patterns are comparatively 'ruled' reinforces the argument that it is the syntagmatic component, as distinct from the paradigmatic one, that gives English its relative stability.

'Jabberwocky' relies heavily on neologism, but neologisms are more varied than the etymological derivation – 'new word' – suggests. Not only is the term 'word' rather fuzzy at the edges, but the epithet 'new' is multifaceted. Words may be variable in *form* (pronounced or written) and, more elusively, in *meaning*, which depends a lot on context and purpose. The newish neologism 'iff', for instance, is pronounced (when spoken at all) the same as 'if'. It seems to occur only in the context of logic, where it always means 'if and only if' (and can be written 'unspeakably' as $\equiv$). But such a strictly limited neolog is exceptionally precise.

Some of Carroll's novelties look quite arbitrary. (One is reminded of Browning's obscure 'Sordello' poem. When asked about the meanings of some of his lines, the poet is said to have explained: 'When I wrote that, only God and Robert Browning knew what it meant; now only God knows.') Rather similarly, Goethe, when asked which of two possible interpretations of an early poem was correct, is reported to have given an equally unhelpful answer. Presumably in German, he forestalled by a couple of centuries a trendy English cliché – 'After all, why not?' The fourth *Supplement* to the *OED* reports Carroll's fanciful derivation of his 'wabe' from the verb to swab or soak because 'the side of a hill' was soaked by the rain. Somewhat more plausibly, 'slithy' was acknowledged to be a blend of 'slimy' and 'lithe'. One linguist has hazarded a guess that 'toves' combined the ends of '*t*urtle d*oves*'. Perhaps more persuasively, he derived 'brillig' from '*bril*liant' and '*ligh*ted', though that theory offended phonological likelihood and rejected Carroll's own perverse definition of his coinage as 'the time of broiling dinner; i.e. the close of the afternoon'. James Thurber (whose home, at least in fiction, was the town of Semantics, Ohio!) wrote a piece with the title 'What Do You Mean, It Was Brillig?' He did not endow 'brillig' with an explanation, but hinted obliquely at verbal possibilities by reporting the malapropisms of his coloured servant, Della. She defied dictionary definitions; she had a brother who, when the First World War ended with an 'Armitrage', got employment burning 'refuge' in an incinerator. In 'The Black Magic of Barney Haller', Thurber's 'I' barked suddenly: 'Listen! Did you know that even when it isn't brillig I can produce slithy toves? Did you happen to know that the mome rath never lived that could outgrabe me . . . ?' Though 'Jabberwocky' is obviously written in English, the '-ig' suffix of 'brillig' is an un-English form suggestive of German – in fact the word survives unchanged in the German translation ('Es brillig war . . .').

Carroll uses an English that, though not strictly nonsensical, is 'garbled'. To 'garble' is, according to the dictionary to 'misrepresent, falsify, mangle, or mutilate'. The immortal Hyman Kaplan, created by the American Leo Rosten (1968; 1970), belonged to a beginner's class in a night school for immigrant adults. His extraordinary use of English, mutilated in its grammar, spelling and punctuation ('Vun mistake on top de odder'), delights us readers but reduces his teacher to utter desperation. Stanley Unwin's Angloid is a different kind of 'mutilation', distorting familiar words into inappropriate related forms:

> all languishing [languages] have a very high redundaload faction [redundancy factor], so that even though the world of mouth is twisty and false, with many a slip twixt club and limp, nevertheless is that does not needly preventilate us from grasping at a crow . . .

The stem of that same 'languishing' was used in a small book, long out of print, entitled *Anguish Languish* (1956). The American author, Howard L. Chace, translated well-known 'NoisierRams' (such as 'Marry Hatter Ladle Limb', 'Sinker Sucker Socks Pants' and 'Oiled Murder Harbored') and 'Furry Tells' ('Ladle Rat Rotten Hut', 'Guilty Looks Enter Tree Beers', 'Center Alley') into his own 'garbled' language. Partly because the stories are very familiar – when read aloud (preferably with an American accent) – the echoes summon up the already well-known words, they are quickly understood, even by speakers of English as a second language (the fables being internationally recognized).

The author's ingenuity allows him to ignore normal word separability. At the simplest level, his three words for the traditional launching of fairy tales – 'Wants pawn term' – represent the four-word equivalent formula. And when Red Riding Hood went into her grandmother's 'cordage', she 'ranker doughbell' and 'entity bet rum'. The 'mural' of her tale is more difficult. The meaning of 'sorghum' (a kind of tropical grass better known to Americans than to Britishers) is totally irrelevant, but its sound helps the listener to unravel the sensible advice to young girls: 'Yonder nor sorghum stenches shut ladle gulls stopper torque wet strainers'.

Obviously, successful communication depends on comprehending both forms and intended meanings, that is, on a balancing-act between medium and message. In *Anguish Languish*, for example, the fact that the message is already possessed by the receiver tolerates the garbling of every word of the medium. A converse balancing situation would apply when the message contained more of the 'now-new' than of the 'old-known'. In that case, the medium would need to be much more orthodox. Consider a couple of sentences not taken from any familiar text but for the moment presented without context:

> Crashes! Water larder warts sunned lack itch udder! Effervescent further deferent saturations an witch way harem, wade heifer haliver tam sang witch worse witch.

For the average reader and probably many others this utterance remains baffling until clues are provided. Given that it is written in the 'anguish languish' (actually in Chace's Introduction), that it should be read aloud with an American accent, that it could be a statement in ordinary English prose, that it says something about words and meanings, and so on, its meaning emerges in the course of appreciating the clues. The utterance is really equivalent to:

> Gracious! What a lot of words sound like each other! If it wasn't for the different situations in which we hear them, we'd have a hell of a time saying which was which.

A final demonstration from Chace's book is its reminder of what primary teachers of reading know well enough, that illustrations can themselves offer invaluable clues to meaning. The picture of a worm confronted by a hungry-looking bird rescues the proverbial sense of their exchange:

> *Worm*:   'Europe oily disk moaning!'
> *Bird*:   'Doily board cashes or warm.'

The volume's frontispiece is masterly, pinpointing the potential anti-social or anti-domesticating effects of the popular 'box'. The picture is of a housewife relaxing in an armchair, enjoying chocolates and a drink, and watching a television programme. An idle vacuum cleaner stands near a door through which we catch sight of a washing-up sink full of crockery vainly awaiting attention. Underneath the picture, the caption reads:

HORSE WAIF ENJOIN TOIL-EVASION

Many other sources of 'productive' deviant English could be explored. Examples can be found in Orwell's Newspeak and other doublespeaks, in unintentionally odd English, in political language, in neologisms, in parodies, in journalism of all sorts. My favourites include:

1 The Swiss conductor who, rebuking an audience unappreciative of his orchestra's performance, barked: 'Don't spoke! Don't spoke! If you didn't like it, you went.'

2 Pedro Carolino, who – in his *New Guide of the Conversation in Portuguese and English* (1836) – gave advice on riding (For to Ride a Horse). A characteristic sentence is: 'Go us more fast never was I seen so much bad beast; she will not nor to bring forward neither put back.'

3 The pseudo-malapropisms used by an American politician to destroy his opponent's chances without being overtly slanderous:

> Are you not aware that Claude Pepper is known all over Washington as a shameless extrovert? Not only that, but this man is reliably reported to practice nepotism with his sister-in-law, and he has a sister who was once a thespian in wicked New York. Worst of all, it is an established fact that Mr Pepper, before his marriage, practiced celibacy.

4 Paul Jennings's 'Fraudian slips', ostensibly taken from the *Grauniad*, the *Tomes* and the *Obsurder*.

5 The Freaky Fable (in *Punch*) which ended with the moral injunction: 'Always be snivel when squeaking to loyalty.'

6 Neologisms such as 'to yomp' (Falklands War language embracing tramping, humping and plodging) and physicists' terminology ('isospin', 'Xenon', 'winos', 'quarks', and even 'charms' and 'naked bottoms').

7 Pre-neologistic descriptions, such as 'The horseless carriage took off in a cloud of smoke and rode on a cushion of air', referring to the invention before the word 'hovercraft' had been devised.

8 The broom that once through Sarah's halls
    In hole and corner sped
Now useless leans 'gainst Sarah's walls
    And gathers dust instead.

Without extending the list, one can surely agree that 'One interesting way of investigating what English *is*, is to study marginal varieties or limiting cases of English' (Stubbs, in Carter, 1982, p. 150).

5 Creativity

> The view of language as 'rule-governed creativity' is especially to be welcomed . . .
>
> (Michael Halliday)

Poetic language

A late sixteenth-century Spanish physician noticed – what has become increasingly obvious – that 'Normal human minds are such that . . . without the help of anybody, they will produce 1000 [sentences] they never heard spoke of . . . inventing and saying such things as they never heard from their masters, nor any mouth' (Huarte de San Juan, quoted in Fromkin and Rodman, 1978, p. 209). According to Chomsky, Huarte distinguished between 'docile wit' and normal intelligence which, 'with its full generative capacities, is the distinction between beast and man'. A disability which restricts a human to a docile wit makes him resemble – in Huarte's words – 'eunuchs, incapable of generation'. On this basis, Chomsky (1966, pp. 78–80) identifies productivity as 'the *creative* aspect of language use' (emphasis added). He offers a sentence – 'Language never gives bilious elephants food for thought' – to represent utterances that we repeatedly hear and understand though we have never heard them before. He argues, refuting Skinner's behaviouristic views, that

> the normal use of language is innovative, in the sense that much of what we say in the course of normal language is entirely new [and what is more] the normal use of language is not only innovative and potentially infinite in scope, but also free from the control of detectable stimuli, either external or internal. (Chomsky, 1968, pp. 11–12)

It follows that language use in these terms is normally productive and can be creative.

There is no clear-cut line separating productivity from creativity. The most creative language is generally assumed to be found in poetry, at least in good poetry. Whoever pronounced that *all* poetry is deviant language was exaggerating, perhaps by concentrating on prototypical poetry such as uses words unconventionally to convey unusually imaginative insights. In this sense, 'verse is "organized violence" committed on everyday language' (Warren and Wellek, 1949, p. 173). But verse, though commonly distinguishing a *formal* characteristic of poetry, is not necessarily *poetic*. Hence the broadest interpretation of 'poetry' in general embraces work ranging from the banal undeviant versifying of Ella Wheeler Wilcox and tombstone epitaphs to the most experimental 'vers libre' defying lexicography and syntax.

Extremes are a bit easier to classify than the more moderate or less eccentric utterances that occur in between. 'Nonsense verse' such as 'Jabberwocky' could have been dealt with under 'creativity' instead of as an example of 'productive' deviance (Chapter 4). James Joyce's prose further blurs the distinction; a Joyce sentence reminding us of this was quoted in a recent newspaper article cleverly titled 'Worderful wondplay':

> To stirr up love's young fizz I tilt with this bridle's cup champagne, dimming douce from her prepair of hide-seeks tight squeezed on my snowybreasted pearlies in their sparkling wisdom nippling her bubblets . . . (the *Guardian*, 17 December 1988)

Here the 'ordinary' meaning is transmitted with 'extraordinary' clarity by a combination of suggestiveness (in both senses), mild neologisms (stirr, prepair, nippling, etc.), and above all a word-dancing rhythm. The language is 'drunk-tilted and effervescent', ambivalently poetic prose or prosaic poetry. On the other hand, because modern English is essentially an uninflected word-order language, there are severe restraints on syntactical deviance, even in the most poetic poetry. The simple single words of Milton's '–him who disobeyes,/Mee disobeyes' (*Paradise Lost*, Book V, lines 611–12) can fail to communicate clearly to young readers because the unconventional word order obscures the intended deictic meaning ('Me' being God, 'him' being Christ). Probably the Latinate mode of thinking, reflected in Latin inflexional forms, caused the poet to underrate the potential ambiguity in English.

Conceptions of 'creativity' and 'creative' have been devalued through excessive exploitation by those attaching more significance to forms than to substance. Scott Fitzgerald wrote in *The Great Gatsby* of 'that flabby impressionality which is dignified under the name of the "creative temperament"'. Robert Frost mockingly compared the writing of so-called free verse to 'playing tennis with the net down'. Bruner (quoted in Richmond, 1967, p. 39) commented that 'The road to banality is paved with creative intentions'. But these criticisms can be dismissed as condemning the *abuse* of creativity. The *legitimate* use is defended by Philip Sidney's famous rhetorical question, in his *Defence of Poesie*: 'But what, shal the abuse of a thing, make the right use odious?'

As an example of obvious creativity in poetic language most people would probably include that of Dylan Thomas for his inventive verbal collocations, as in 'once below a time', 'a grief ago', 'all the sun long', 'heron-priested shore'. Leech has set the very normal 'broad smile' against 'free smile', 'damp smile', and – most deviantly – 'high smile'. More sizeable examples are Thomas's 'What sixth of wind blew out the burning gentry', Emily Dickinson's 'And then he drank a dew / From a convenient grass', Edith Sitwell's 'fruitbuds that whimper' and James Britton's wry, 'pun-governed' lines about an 'ageing schoolmaster', *One is Company* (quoted in Meek and Miller, 1984):

> And still in the dark sat he,
> Sighing, 'Leave me alone,' to the leaves that were blown
> From the boughs of a sycamore tree.
>   And they leaved him alone:
>   And they leaved him right over.

The late Philip Larkin wrote poetry that approached everyday personal concerns as closely as possible. His 'Church Going' was made memorable by cycle-clips:

> Hatless, I take off
> My cycle-clips in awkward reverence.

More profoundly, he wonders whether the very last visitor to 'this accoutred frowsty barn', before it finally decays, might be 'Some ruin-bibber, randy for antique'. The same ambivalent detachment is captured in another of his poems, in which – feeling a mixture of superiority and envy – he watches through a window a convivial dance:

> But not for me, nor I for them; and so
> With happiness. Therefore I stay outside,
> Believing this; and they maul to and fro,
> Believing that; and both are satisfied,
> If no one has misjudged himself. Or lied.

> (quoted in the *Times Literary Supplement*, 18 May 1956)

Craig Raine (who incidentally has contributed to sound recordings of Larkin's poems) also takes his topics from ordinary life. But he seeks – in his own words – to 'defamiliarize the familiar world'. The titles of some of his poems indicate the ordinariness, occasionally the earthiness, of some of his starting-points – 'City Gent', 'Words on the Page', 'Baize Doors', 'In Modern Dress', 'Arsehole'. He has explained that Forster's epigraph to *Abinger Harvest* ironically reduces Saint George, killer of the dragon, to the less heroic status of one who 'wore a top-hat once' and had been an army contractor supplying 'indifferent bacon' to the troops. Raine reduces the myth by choosing a profession which 'some people thought humdrum' and bringing out its potential poetry. His poem 'The Butcher' emphasizes how a Rotary Club butcher, usually serving in a shop full of housewives, enjoys a feeling of licence and innuendo induced by his familiarity with nudity, with breasts, buttocks and loins. Similarly, in his well-known clever lines on 'A Martian Sends a Postcard Home', he creates a strange world out of a commonplace one. He 'defamiliarizes' not only the postcard, which is explicitly named as such, but also homely objects presented unnamed in riddles which can be semantically disentangled from the words. These items include 'Caxtons', which are mechanical birds with many wings, and some of which are 'treasured with their markings', 'time tied to the wrist', and a 'haunted apparatus' which sleeps, snores when it is picked up, cries, is carried to the lips and soothed, but can be awakened deliberately by tickling with a finger.

Anglo-Saxon riddles qualify as literature. But all riddling is not *ipso facto* literary just because literary creations can be cast in riddle form. Raine's riddles occupy a kind of no man's land. Some critics judge them as ingenious verbal tricks exploiting analogies. Others judge them as creatively imaginative metaphors. Analogy and figurative language are to be found in the same marginal territory. It is a naïve assumption, shared apparently by some teachers, that figures of speech belong exclusively or predominantly to literature. In reality, they are elements in rhetoric, and modern rhetoric is closely equivalent to verbal (not just oral) composition. Such misconception as exists probably derives from a specious separation of language from literature. However convenient such a separation is for the organization of educational institutions, for examination boards and for the qualifications awarded, it remains logically, philosophically and academically invalid. A recent complaint, by an English specialist (Clout, 1987, p. 35) deplored 'the curious but persistent belief cultivated among extremists on both sides of a quite illusory barricade – that the academic studies of language and of literature are mutually exclusive'.

Obviously all literature is language. The important difference between literary and non-literary language is a qualitative one. Raine's explicit objective (implicit in much other poetry) of defamiliarizing the ordinary world uses the same key-word as Roman Jakobson used in explaining his 'communicative model'. Griffith (1987) reproduces that famous linguist's diagram of 'Functions in a speech event' (Jakobson, 1960):

referential

poetic

emotive ———————————————————————————————— conative

phatic

metalingual

Griffith's gloss argues that 'Jakobson was thinking primarily of lyric poetry . . . But Jakobson was also writing as an inheritor of Russian formalism, in which the literariness of literature consisted precisely of the way in which it *defamiliarized the language*, making its audience aware of the constructed nature of what it was reading, so that *the medium was no longer transparent*' (Griffith, 1987, pp. 3–4, emphasis added).

The transparent-opaque distinction has proved particularly useful in schematizing language use. An 'illusory barricade' separating language from literature is contradicted by the fact that ordinary, routine, non-literary language succeeds to the extent that it lets meaning through with minimal consciousness of language as such, whereas literary language conspicuously and deliberately draws attention to its linguistic self. In the terminology used by Britton, the opaque stained-glass *poetic* language adopts the role of spectator, while, at the opposite end of his continuum, transactional language in the role of participant corresponds to clear glass.

Literal or metaphorical

Growing interest in semantics has brought with it in the last few decades a serious study of figurative language, producing titles such as *A Study of Metaphor* (Mooij, 1976), *Metaphor and Thought* (Ortony, 1979) and *Metaphors We Live By* (Lakoff and Johnson, 1980). Teachers of English sometimes interpret 'metaphor' narrowly, contrasting it with simile, personification, etc. as one of a set of figures of speech and treating it as mainly or exclusively a feature of poetic and literary language. Setting figurative language in general against literal language is broader and more satisfactory, except that it raises questions about what and how rare are strictly literal words. Ortony (1979, p. 3) employs a more esoteric term with fewer variable connotations when he generalizes that 'all language is tropological'. Originally a rhetorical 'trope' in Latin meant 'a figure of speech which consists in the use of a word or phrase in a sense other than that which is proper to it' (*Shorter Oxford English Dictionary*), but evolution and linguistic change have abandoned the difficult, outmoded sense of 'proper' (cf. propriety in language use). 'Speaking by tropes' has become equivalent to using figurative language, or, in the largest sense, metaphor. Consequently, Lakoff and Johnson are able to argue that most language is metaphorical. Not only, in their view, does metaphor pervade our language, but 'the human conceptual system is metaphorically structured and defined. Metaphors as linguistic expressions are possible precisely because there are metaphors in a person's conceptual system' (Lakoff and Johnson, 1980, p. 6). Hugh R. Walpole (1941, p. 154) deplores a misconception that metaphors belong specially to literature: 'Some of our literary professors have misled us about Metaphor. It is not an extra beauty stuck on to language – it is language'. Perhaps, as Trevor Griffiths is supposed to have said, 'There's more metaphor in Manchester than in Middlemarch.'

As with most language distinctions, that between the literal and the metaphorical is fuzzy. Derrida's *Of Grammatology*, translated into English in 1974 and referred to in the Kingman Report (DES, 1988, para. 2.25), claims that 'the precision and exactitude of language' exists above all in literalness [*propriété*] and should be absolutely universal and literal [*propre*], i.e. non-metaphorical' (Derrida, 1974, p. 27). Doubts about what Derrida really means – or what his translator seems to make him mean – namely, that in language-use literalness equals propriety or properness, are bolstered by dictionary definitions. The relevant equivalence of *propriété* in Larousse is 'Convenance exacte d'un mot, d'un terme, à l'idée à exprimer' but *convenance* is defined as 'conformité, i.e. qualité de ce qui convient, est approprié'. The notion of 'appropriateness' is – at least in English usage – opposed to, rather than equated with, the idea of 'proper' usage or 'correctness'.

When Richards (1938, p. 118) considered the relationship between literal and metaphorical meanings, he recognized that, even with the simplest words – such as 'leg' – the boundary between literal and metaphorical is not fixed or reliable:

To what do we apply it literally? A horse has legs literally, so has a spider, but how about a chimpanzee? Has it two legs or four? And how about a star-fish? Has it arms or legs or neither? And, when a man has a wooden leg, is it a metaphoric or a literal leg? The answer to this last is that it is both. It is literal in one set of respects, metaphoric in another. A word may be simultaneously both literal and metaphoric.

Whether or not the 'both' solution is reasonable, Richards's view is in principle consistent with the fact that language is, as we might expect, essentially homocentric, so that the human limb is literally named 'leg', but the same term is extended analogically and metaphorically to similar limbs. Metaphor involves understanding one kind of thing in terms of another. But, there being many more 'other' things than the original 'one', it follows that many more of the meanings of polysemic words are metaphorical than the single literal meaning. This supports Widdowson's (1979, p. 142) broader argument that

metaphor surely lies at the heart of everyday communicative behaviour. What seems to be abnormal is *non*-metaphorical communication, a strict conformity to rules. Indeed, if language users were strict conformists, their language would presumably lose its capacity for adaption and gradually fossilize.

The best-known language which tries to eliminate metaphor is Orwell's Newspeak in *Nineteen Eighty-Four*. The Newspeak Dictionary that was being devised would allow each word only one meaning, the basic literal one. Rigid definition of 'free', for example, would restrict it to the meaning in 'free from lice' or 'free from weeds'. A 'rat' would refer only to the familiar rodent and not be extendable to treacherous men. Oddly – in the real world inevitably – Syme, Orwell's director of the pruning project intended drastically to simplify vocabulary, explained in *metaphorical* Oldspeak that his objective was that of 'cutting the language down to the bone'. In any case, the intention was, by shrinking word meanings, to eliminate unacceptable thought and make 'thoughtcrime' impossible. In effect, such a language would not only be politically objectionable but would condemn itself to sterility and fossilization.

It must be conceded, however, that language – if it is to survive – needs constant renewal of its metaphorical resources. 'Most lexical items', we are told, 'prove to be dead metaphors that were alive and kicking at some time in the past' (Sadock, in Ortony 1979, p. 48). According to Goldberg (1938, p. 76), Jespersen described language as 'a cemetery of dead metaphors'. A 'taste of history' has lost any analogical gustatory sense it may once have had and a 'shotgun' wedding no longer evokes the vision of an armed father-in-law. Mooij (1976, pp. 123–4) contends that 'power', 'current', 'wave' and similar terms used in natural science were necessary and useful metaphors which in the course of time have developed into new literal terms homonymous with the original forms. The idea of 'developing in time' reminds us that 'literal', like most adjectives, is temporally gradient. The word 'death', used non-literally as in 'dead metaphor', tends to obscure the 'more or less' flexibility of figurative death. Literal death is – leaving aside recent developments distinguishing brain-death from biological death –

absolute, but metaphorical death varies relatively from extinct, through dormant, to active. The terminology used by the Kingman Report's model (DES, 1988, p. 19, Box 3) contrasts *frozen* metaphors – such as 'kick the bucket', where the literal sense has vanished – with *productive* metaphors – such as, 'run out of time', in which the figurative life still survives.

A further caution has to be exercised with the analogical nature of much figurative language. There is nothing creative in the sort of arithmetical analogies that once flourished in intelligence tests popular with education authorities. The symbols employed in an item such as:

As 3 : 9 so is 4 : (16)

are clear-cut within the decimal system. The verbal symbols in

As HAND is to WRIST so is FOOT to (ANKLE)

are almost as reliable (and unimaginative). But the metaphorical analogy intrinsic to a popular advertisement is – or at least was in its first years – distinctly creative and therefore less than absolutely reliable. The thought process which could be represented as follows –

As POWER is to TIGER so is PETROL to CAR

– produced 'Put a tiger in your tank'. Commercial slogans such as this are intended, in order to promote sales, to be clear and unambiguous, but here linguistic inventiveness may well have proved confusing. Did it persuade drivers to put into their tanks one brand of petrol rather than the others? Or did it encourage drivers to feel as if they were 'roaring away'? Or, less plausibly, did it induce drivers to fill up whenever a favoured petrol-pump occurred?

This same figure of speech illustrates the capacity of metaphor to extend across language domains and registers, from advertisements to techniques of image-making and thence to literature. In Muriel Spark's novel, significantly called *The Public Image*, the soi-disant film actress Annabel Christopher is described by her husband as 'a twentieth-century Jane Eyre', a 'tiger in the tank' combining 'the effect of external propriety with a tiger in her soul'. The manipulating power of film publicity allows her Italian director to impose a simulacrum of personality and acting talent on 'an English girl from Wakefield, with a peaky face and mousey hair'. Billed first as an 'English Lady-Tiger', she is then transformed into 'The Cat-Tiger'.

A metaphorical use can expand not only to serve a wide range of language domains, but also to transcend inter-language barriers. When very tall multi-storey buildings first came to dominate the skyscape, most conspicuously in the USA, an English-speaking observer created the 'skyscraper' metaphor. As the concrete things multiplied internationally, the verbalization expressing the concept was adopted internationally, yielding German 'Wolkenkratzer', French 'gratte-ciel', Italian 'grattacielo' and Spanish 'rascacielo'.

Traditional notions of metaphor focus inadequately on linguistic surfaces,

neglecting deeper conceptual implications. The skyscraping analogy has probably lost most of its metaphorical force, but the fact that particular metaphors fade
and die is not evidence of more general decay. Rather it is testimony to their initial
success and to the need for constant renewal of metaphorical strength.
Metaphor, in short, is not purely decorative or additional. Ortony (1979, p. 2)
compromises by presenting 'two alternative approaches to metaphor as an
essential characteristic of the creativity of language; and metaphor as deviant and
parasitic upon normal usage'. If 'normal usage' is judged qualitatively, in terms of
the importance and human value of communication rather than – as apparently
by Ortony – in terms of sheer, often trivial, frequency of utterance, we can accept
Huizinga's (1935, p. 37) conclusion that 'Without metaphor the handling of
general concepts such as culture and civilization become impossible'. We may be
able, further, to agree with Steiner (1975) that:

> Ambiguity, polysemy, opaqueness, the violation of grammatical and logical se-
> quences, reciprocal incomprehensions, the capacity to lie – these are not pathologies
> of language but the roots of its genius. Without them the individual and the species
> would have withered.

It is worthwhile, indeed necessary, to tolerate these deviant features in order to
reap the rewards of language's creativity.

6 Stability and change

> Stability in language is synonymous with *rigor mortis*.
>
> (Ernest Weekley)

Language and thought

The relationship of language to thought is as puzzling as it is important. Questions about knowing and saying have sought answers from people of all ages and capacities. We are often told that a little girl, warned to 'Think before you speak!', responded with a question of great relevance to educators: 'How do I know what I think until I hear what I say?' (see, for example, Gatherer, 1980, p. 48). Virtually the same question has been attributed to 'an old lady', to E. M. Forster, to Auden, and doubtless to many others. The implied answer to this quasi-rhetorical question is that language is assumed to be essential for thinking. Nevertheless, some thinkers have asserted the contrary. Bishop Berkeley found that words so hindered thinking that he tried to keep them out of his thoughts. Francis Galton sought in his thinking to 'disembarrass it of words' (Harding, 1967, p. 89). Coleridge (1884, pp. 311–12) speculated that

> processes of thought might be carried on independent and apart from spoken or written language. I do not in the least doubt if language had been denied or withheld from man, or that he had not discovered or improved that mode of intercommunication, thought, as thought, would have been a process more simple, more easy, and more perfect than the present, and would have both included and evolved other and better means for its own manifestations, than any that exist now.

Thought being 'beyond' language, its mysteries can only be hinted at obliquely, often by metaphors. Some behaviourists described thinking as subvocalizing or 'merely talking, but talking with concealed musculature' (quoted from J. B. Watson by Dinneen, 1967, p. 263). Sapir (1921, p. 223) believed that 'thought is nothing but language denuded of its outward garb'. Vigotsky (1961, p. 514) more cautiously argued that 'Thought is not expressed in words, but comes into existence through them'.

In so far as language expresses rational thought, the study of language is necessarily involved in the study of the rational mind. For philosophers, taking all knowledge to be their province, language served the 'need to discover a logic, a foundation of certitude upon which to rest their arguments and investigations' (Land, 1986, p. 237). Unlike Keats, whose 'Negative Capability' meant 'capable of being in uncertainties, philosophers have striven to make up their minds about everything' (Tsur, 1975, p. 776). Francis Bacon observed human lust for order and commented:

> The human understanding, from its peculiar nature, easily supposes a greater degree of order and equality in things than it really finds; and although many things in nature be *sui generis* and most irregular, will yet invent parallels and conjugates and relatives, where no such thing is. (Bacon 1971, p. 391)

The inherent dilemma was recognized in ancient Greece. It caused disagreement about the nature of the world itself. In opposition to those like Parmenides who regarded the universe as spherical, unchanging and indivisible, Heraclitus ('the weeping philosopher') maintained that all things were in a state of flux, the external world being in a harmonious process of constant change. A fluid world inevitably produces new things to say and therefore needs a new and changing language with which to think (*pace* Berkeley, Galton, etc.), to express and to communicate.

The doctrine of Heraclitus caused much alarm by contradicting the universal assumption that reality was stable and fixed. Though linguistic evidence since his day has accumulated to demonstrate that language changes, the lust for certainty, guaranteeing stability and security, has resisted acceptance of linguistic and semantic change. The central paradox has been illustrated by Hockett's (1968, p. 85) analogy with the movement of a clock's hands:

> either the hand moves steadily and slowly, or else it moves in individual jerks so small that they are indetectable to the naked eye. But – to the naked eye – there is no significant difference between these two possibilities. This is exactly the kind of conclusion we are forced to reach about linguistic change. It is in this way that a language can be, at any one time – for an observer or for its users – a stable system, and yet be constantly changing.

A recent description of the paradoxical dilemma accepts that language change is both normal and disturbing:

> Rather than taking situations of flux, change, and heterogeneity as exceptions, there may be value in taking them as the norm, for underneath the 'fixed' language of times of stability there has always been repressed variation, for example regional and class dialects, in greater or less contact . . . Yet change causes uncertainty, anxiety, so that with awareness of variation there can arise a desire for order, for just those synchronic structures found in more 'static' societies. The effect seems to be that the very means of recording language and thus making language change, are drawn on to defend language stability and to mask change as mere 'deviance'. (Bourne, 1988, pp. 92–3)

Obviously a lot depends critically on the rate of change in relation to the span of human lifetime. The mathematician-philosopher A. N. Whitehead (1933) surveyed the long history of civilization. Taking the risk of oversimplifying, he made large generalizations about 'the recent shortening of the time-span between notable changes in social customs', estimating the periods of time needed for humans to adjust to new developments. Paraphrasing his data and putting his round numbers in tabular form:

(a) gradual changes of physical configuration (for example, by the elevation of mountains) needed periods of the order of a million years;

(b) gradual changes of climate took about 5000 years;

(c) regional overpopulations needed about 500 years to be recognized;

(d) new technologies (such as the chipping of flints, the invention of fire, the taming of animals, the development of metallurgy) also used up about 500 years;

(e) great advances consequent upon, for example, the invention of gunpowder, printing, expertise in navigation occupied about 300 years (from about 1400 to 1700);

(f) modern developments (for example, steam power, machinery) needed only about two generations (1830–90).

Details of analysis and dating are less important than the accelerating pace of accommodating to novelties. Whitehead's most significant conclusion was that in the past the time-span of important change was considerably longer than that of a single human life. Thus mankind was trained to adapt to fixed conditions. Today this time-span is considerably shorter than that of human life, and accordingly our training must prepare individuals to face novel conditions (Whitehead, 1933, p. 118).

The relevance of this argument for teaching is that the traditions extending from the age of Plato (fifth century BC) to the end of the nineteenth century included traditional doctrines of education which involved 'the vicious assumption that each generation will substantially live amid the conditions governing the lives of its children. We are living in the first period of human history for which this assumption is false' (Whitehead, 1933, p. 117). The further relevance of this state of affairs to language teaching is that the tradition was maintained essentially by verbal transmission. It was taken for granted that a stable society was one disciplined by rules – moral, social and political – formulated in a 'ruled' language. Such an authoritarian language was established by 'two influential minorities, the grammarians and the writers, both groups belonging to an educational élite. It was in the interests of both to inculcate a concern for 'correct' usage and to agree on what 'correct' usage should be . . . On the whole they were favoured by social stability, political unification and strong government' (Harris, 1987, p. 105).

The great changes enumerated by Whitehead proved irresistible. His list – (a)–(f) above – proceeded from revolutions in geography and climate physically beyond human control and from overpopulation realistically uncontrollable, through technological changes so advantageous as not to invite control, to inventions and developments that attracted such minor resistance as could be dismissed as Luddite opposition to progress. History seems to support two conflicting factors: that language always changes, but that many people always try to stop it changing. The beliefs that motivate the latter include, as well as the already mentioned lust for certainty, convictions that linguistic change is wrong, that a changing language is unstable, that an unstable language prevents clear and exact communication, that unconventional usage is unacceptable, and that mistakes in speech and writing are deplorable. In any absolute or total sense, these latter beliefs are obviously untenable. Everything depends on the relative degree of conviction with which they are held.

Many such views are *unthought* beliefs and assumptions, based probably on resistance to serious, rational thought itself. William Cowper, according to Jeffreys (1955, p. 11), encapsulated reluctance to undertake thinking in his reference to 'the insupportable fatigue of thought'. Obstinate resistance to contemplating curriculum reform in a (fictional) palaeolithic age induced self-destruction of the tigers in the parable of *The Saber-Toothed Curriculum*: 'Then, as now, there were few lengths to which men would not go to avoid the labor and pain of thought' (Peddiwell, 1939, p. 25).

Bertrand Russell goes devastatingly further by blaming fear more than fatigue:

> Men fear thought as they fear nothing else on earth – more than ruin, more even than death. Thought is subversive and revolutionary, destructive and terrible; thought is merciless to privilege, established institutions and comfortable habits; thought is anarchic and lawless, indifferent to authority, careless of the well-tried wisdom of the ages. Thought looks into the pit of hell and is not afraid. (quoted in Randall, 1976, p. 680)

This may be provocatively overstated, but it is difficult to deny that 'comfortable habits' prefer the familiar and the recognizable status quo to the disturbances caused by change and unpredictability. Nevertheless, one major function of education is to foster criticism. Blamires (1950, p. 87) argued persuasively that 'in regard to contemporary life one function of education is the dissemination of discontent'.

The outstanding exemplar of a language thought to be as near to perfection as humanly possible has long been classical Greek. Its perfection guaranteed lasting and unchanging stability. But classical Greek was artificial in the sense that it was a language 'of great artifice'. By contrast, as Frege is reported as saying, 'natural language is rife with vagueness, ambiguity, lack of logical perspicuity, and, indeed, logical coherence' (Baker and Hacker, 1984, p. 37). It is the *spoken* Greek language that has changed since the centuries of the 'Golden Age' and has been accused of deterioration. Modern written Greek language has also changed, but classical writings have, of course, been preserved in books. It is primarily speaking, however, that ensures the lasting life of a language. The great majority of the world's languages exist only as speech. The death of a spoken language is usually caused, not by inherent obsolescence, but by the death or disappearance of its speakers.

A problem that cannot reasonably be debated in terms of absolute versus relative considerations turns into a question of how much stability a language needs for survival and how much change it can tolerate. Speakers of different languages make different assessments about proportions of stability and change. Educational corollaries involve judgements about speech education, about how much speaking by children should be tolerated or encouraged at school and in the home, how much 'interference' by teachers should be allowed, recommended or required, and so on. At an international conference on mother-tongue teaching – held in 1979 at Hamburg's Unesco Institute for Education – clashes occurred in evaluations of spoken and written language. A representative from France reported that:

> The written language has been considered as the sole frame of reference, the living, spoken language consequently being felt to be only rough, a language incomplete and incorrect. The one system has become inferior in value to the other.

As a result, she continued, with obvious disapproval:

> In education, this difference in value between the two systems resulted in the unreasonable demand that the child should express himself orally according to the style of written language. (Canham, 1972, p. 78)

In Britain, comparable 'appreciation' (up-pricing) of written English and depreciation (down-pricing) of spoken English are expressed by the conservative Queen's English Society and the Conservative Party's Centre for Policy Studies. Sheila Lawlor, a leading official of the latter organization, has committed herself to absurd assertions that 'Without knowledge of grammatical terms, pupils are not equipped to form a correct sentence' and that 'There is no reason to imagine that pupils learn from talking' (1988, pp. 22–3 and 18–19).

Such assertions are not supported by reputable evidence. The research and experience of many linguists and teachers offer evidence to the contrary and, fortunately, the National Curriculum Council has insisted – against official pressure – that spoken language should retain the important position recommended in the second Cox Report (DES, 1989). 'Correct' sentences have been written (and spoken) without grammatical knowledge by learners as well as by accomplished users of English. Recognition of the 'primacy of speech' and of the value of talk in negotiating meaning – both among learners and between them and adults – has effectively and without demonstrable loss modified teaching and testing practices. Inevitably, more attention to the spoken word reduces the time spent in schools on writing. But a reduction in the hours of pen-pushing, an excessive proportion of which is often devoted to note-taking, copying, recapitulation and the writing of routine 'essays' (documented in the Inspectorate's

Aspects of Secondary Education in England 1979, Chapter 6) has not devalued the importance of literacy in writing.

Stability needs change

It is not necessary to analyse in more detail the features of stability in language, beyond adding that the 'standstill' argument has turned injunctions to 'do it as the classical Greek and Latin languages did' more and more into 'do it as the prescriptive grammars and the usage handbooks require' and even to follow the *ipsedixitisms* of 'do it *my* way'. The 'fix-it' dogma – do it by fiat – was managed internationally by academies (French, Spanish, Italian, Swedish, Hebrew). Attempts to set up similar institutions in Germany and the United States failed. In England the failures of Defoe and Swift to mobilize support have been thoroughly recorded. Defoe thought it should be made as criminal to coin words without the authority of his proposed academy as to forge coins. In 1712 Swift addressed his well-known *Proposal for Correcting, Improving and Ascertaining the English Tongue* to the Lord High Treasurer of Great Britain. Swift's academy was to 'fix our language for ever'. The strength of his personal conviction and its inherent fallacy were contained in his opinion that 'it is better a Language should not be wholly perfect, than that it should be perpetually changing' (*Proposal*, p. 31). Roman grammarians commenting on the work of classical authors had illustrated their grammatical statements with quotations, not from their contemporaries, but from 'Golden Age' writers such as Cicero and Vergil (Robins, 1951, p. 62). Dr Johnson followed this practice by preferring 'to collect examples for his Dictionary from writers before the reformation, whose works I regard as *the wells of English undefiled*'. He was consequently criticized by Joseph Priestley for preferring the language of the past to that of the then present day (of Addison and indeed of Swift himself). But Johnson was also – and somewhat ambiguously – forward-looking when he acknowledged in his Preface that 'the laws of the life of a language are stronger than any human lawmaker', that actual usage ruled use and that academies of language were futile.

Nevertheless, as lexicography escapes from the 'drudgery' it meant for Johnson to a more influential position, the work of academies is undertaken more modestly by including comments in dictionaries on vexed usages and by employing 'experts' to provide consolidated judgements of word use. In Britain, both the *Oxford Paperback Dictionary* (1979) and the *Oxford Guide to English Usage* (1983) add prescriptive or at least 'judgemental' observations on items of 'divided usage'. The use of 'due to' in such sentences as 'Play was stopped, due to rain', for instance, is ruled by the *Paperback Dictionary* as 'incorrect', while the use of 'due to' as a compound preposition is mildly disapproved in the *Guide* as being 'widely regarded as unacceptable'. A typical example of the employment of 'experts' has been the usage panel paid to advise the *America Heritage Dictionary*. Though John Simon (1981, pp. 6–7), in a book pointedly subtitled 'Reflections on Literacy and its Decline', found severe fault with the membership of that panel, which 'ranges from some persons of impeccable credentials to others from whom you would not want to buy a used car (or a misused verb)', he obstinately went on to express the unrealistic view that 'in this direction salvation must lie: the eventual creation of an Academy of Anglo-American Language'.

The paradox at the heart of the problem was neatly expressed by the young Tancredi in Lampedusa's *The Leopard*: 'If we want things to stay as they are, things will have to change.' Change, in other words, ensures stability – in language as in life. Somewhere between minimum change conducive to stagnation and maximum change leading to chaos there must be optimum change. The popular analogy with a river illustrates the difficulty of describing any optimum state. A river has a high degree of stability in direction, size and speed – but one can never bathe in the same river twice. We are compelled when measuring language phenomena to use a crude, impressionistic, 'dipstick' method. Applying this method to the English language, it is possible more or less to separate out some linguistic features in an order roughly proceeding from shorter, more static written forms (such as spelling) to longer, more elusive semantic 'strings'.

A teacher's attitude towards language use can, in broad terms, be placed on a scale measuring tolerance of change. A ten-point scale, offered by ten Brinke's *The complete mother-tongue curriculum* (1986, p. 172), is shown in Figure 2. Apart from difficulties in defining 'comprehension', 'jargon' and 'standard language' in these three boxes, any one teacher may occupy different points on the scale when judging different language features.

A few specific features – including what DES (1989, para. 17.1) calls 'secretarial' (as distinct from 'composing') aspects – may be considered according to these criteria.

Spelling rituals

Printing invented misspelling. Before then, word spellings enjoyed free variation within the limits of semantic identification, that is, so long as the misspelling did

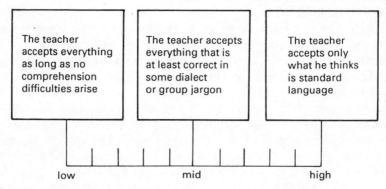

Figure 2   Attitudes to correctness
Derived from ten Brinke (1986, p. 172)

not, in its context, cause misreading as a different word. Post-printing standard-ization was imposed for the convenience of typesetters rather than for purposes of comprehension and communication. That it made for easier and quicker reading and that it removed, especially for second-language learners of English, an unnecessary complication supplementary to the fossilized arbitrariness of our orthography was an incidental advantage. The extraordinary importance attached by employers to conventional spelling owes much to superficial top-dressing respectability. Sadly, some teachers also overweigh 'correct' spelling because of the ease of detection of 'incorrectness'. The inordinate amount of attention given to spelling obeys Thorsten Veblen's (1925, p. 257) law:

> English orthography satisfies all the requirements of the canons of reputability under the law of conspicuous waste. It is archaic, cumbrous, and ineffective; its acquisition consumes much time and effort; failure to acquire it is easy of detection. Therefore it is the first and readiest test of reputability in learning, and conformity to its ritual is indispensable to a blameless scholastic life.

Without advocating a return to 'free trade' in spelling, it is desirable to recognize that, while spelling has become – as a byproduct of printing techniques – 'probably the most immutable part of English' (Veblen, 1925, p. 62), it is not carved in tablets of stone. A poor-spelling university lecturer in English spoke for many well-educated non-spellers when, in a recent letter to the *Guardian*, he expressed his longing to be liberated from 'the bondage of "correct" spelling'.

Jespersen is quoted (Chapman, 1988, p. 39) as referring scathingly to 'that pseudo-historical and anti-educational abomination, the English spelling.' In so far as this 'abomination' is (because it has become) phonetically inaccurate, it follows that misspellings can be more 'really' accurate than conventionally 'correct' spelling. Chapman is able to quote many examples of deliberate misspelling in literature (where it usually aims at representing dialectical speech), in song lyrics (for example, '*Yeah*, right / *C'mon* everybody / On *yer* rocket / Okay, let *'em* in / It's a simple solution, *innit?*) and in advertising (Bar-B-Q, Kwik Save), but points out that any protest can only be made in a literate society that accepts the convention being protested against.

The irregularities of 'normal' English spelling have been exaggerated. Notori-ously '-ough' is pronounced in a number of different ways, but Shaw's possibly ironic 'ghoti' spelling for 'fish' is implausible – an obvious linguistic fact that may have escaped the attention of a linguistically underinformed Shaw. It has been pointed out (for example, by Michael Stubbs, 1980, p. 51) that 'gh' is sounded as 'f' only when it occurs at the end of a morpheme. G. Dewey's similar but more extreme spelling of 'taken' as 'phtheighchound' is doubtless open to similar objections to deriving the graphic from the phonic rather than the other way round. Conventions of spelling have been regular enough to resist for centuries attempts at spelling reform. Proposals for change include: the modified spelling invented and used by Bullokar in his *Bref Grammar* (1586), generally accepted as the earliest vernacular English grammar; seventeenth-century experiments with 'real' and 'universal' characters suitable for recording scientific investigations for Royal Society meetings; the activities of Isaac Pitman (who published his *Phonotypy* in 1844); the Spelling Reform Association (1876); the Simplified Spelling Society (1908); the Society for Pure English (1911); and the proponents of i.t.a. (this last supposedly helping learners to read before transferring to traditional orthography).

The Spelling Reform Association was an American institution, and Americans enjoyed more success in deliberately imposing changes assumed to favour simplicity and consistency. Noah Webster's strong preference for '-or' (as in 'favor') and '-er' (as in 'center') prevailed in America in most words of the kind. Other reforms included the reduction of double consonants ('traveling' and the like) and using 'practice' as both noun and verb (see Crystal, 1987b, pp. 213–17). On the other hand, governmental views by no means always prevailed. President Benjamin Franklin, in a letter 'On Modern Innovations in the English Language and in Printing', written to Webster in 1789, deplored printing practices which, in the interests of uniformity and 'evenness', dropped the long 's' (ʃ), ceased to use capital initial letters to distinguish nouns from verbs, and banished italic type. His own invention of a Reformed Spelling system perhaps deserved its lack of success. He started a letter to Mary (Polly) Stevenson with a sentence in good plain English bizarrely spelled:

> Diir Poli,
> Yii intended to hev sent iu chiz Pepers sunyr, byt biing bizi fargat it. . . .
> (Baron, 1982, p. 72, Figure 2)

President Theodore Roosevelt's proclamation in 1906 ordering the adoption of simplified spelling failed much more completely than a Bill presented to the British Parliament in 1949; the latter was rejected by only a narrow majority. It is significant that a standard American-English spelling has been adopted in Britain for computer *programs*. This development suggests that word-processors will, via their programs, reduce further the small percentage of alternative British-English spellings (such as '-ise'/'-ize', 'judgement'/'judgment', 'adviser'/'advisor').

Teachers' judgements of acceptability in spelling might reasonably be placed in the left-hand box of ten Brinke's Figure 2, using comprehensibility as the main criterion. They would hope to nudge learners towards the standard language right-hand box as they approached school-leaving age. With younger children, presumably expressing simpler thoughts, teachers could be much more tolerant, refraining from such insistence on conventional spelling as to discourage adventurous and creative exploitation of half-learned but less commonplace words. They could allow, and even encourage, interesting neologisms (for example, a 'fiercesome' sight, a 'harduous' task, 'vividity'). On the other hand, they could not be expected to accept all the 209 ways in which 10-year-olds (according to Margaret Peters) spelled 'saucer' (1967, p. 7). Nor could context be expected to rescue 'ssos' in 'Donkeys like *ssos*', using the remarkable spelling of 'thistles' reported by Miss Read (*Village School*, p. 30). A more serious problem is that of 'density' of misspelling. A few, but not the full sequence, of the single-word curiosities could be tolerated in a sentence devised by Frank Smith (1928, p. 181).

> The none tolled hymn she had scene a pare of bear feat inn hour rheum.

This frequency does not prohibit comprehension, but it makes reading excessively irritating.

Peculiarities of punctuation

It is often necessary to distinguish between punctuation by the voice ('pointing' spoken utterance by patterns of intonation) and punctuation by writing (or printing). Spoken punctuation is as old as speech, but written punctuation is not as old as writing. Word separation, unknown until the fifth century BC, was introduced in early Latin inscriptions by dots, then by dots or spaces. It was only in the early Middle Ages that spacing words became the general practice. Some medieval manuscripts apparently used both syllable spacing and word spacing to mark pauses, as if today (according to Bolinger, 1975, p. 472) we might write 'wish ful' and 'dish ful', or

> If you see him when you get home   call me.

In modern times, typewriters have made available a considerable range of punctuation marks and capital letters, but archy, the cockroach created by don marquis (1934), lacked weight and therefore couldn't use the shift key. He relied solely on lower case to produce his life of mehitabel the cat. The growth of literacy emphasized the incompatibility between the two major purposes of punctuation. Rhetorical (or oratorical) punctuation was meant primarily, by marking breath junctures, to help breath control. It was a subsidiary coincidence that enabled it sometimes (but by no means always) also to mark boundaries between syntactic structures. The latter was the main objective of the rival grammatical punctuation, designed formally to mark segmentation into phrases, clauses and sentences for communication in reading and writing. Some of the earliest symbols have not survived. For example, *The Pageant of the Birth, Life and Death of Richard Beauchamp Earl of Warwick*, written towards the end of the fifteenth century, used a system that included the obsolete perioslash (./) and periocomma (:) in addition to the period or full-stop, the comma and the slash (/). The last of these linked sentences, while the perioslash separated groups of conjoined sentences (Arakelian, 1975, p. 614). Printing stabilized punctuation, gradually establishing the system that has become the 'slight' punctuation favoured by the Fowler brothers in their *King's English* (1906, p. 234) and used today.

Our modern punctuation system relies on fewer than a dozen marks, a few of them (. ? !) indicating sentence boundaries, the others (, ; : —) being internal to a sentence. This, compared with musical notation, is comparatively crude. On the other hand, it is so simple as to leave little scope for change. Noticeable tendencies favour shorter sentences and therefore more full stops (both bare 'periods' and the base dots used in question and exclamation marks). Those conservatives who would prefer what is already a very stable feature to be made rigidly prescriptive sometimes deplore the apparent decline of the semicolon, which has been called 'the master stop of literary prose'. Powell (1976) has argued that 'once dull language has invaded the novel, dull punctuation follows'; he could remember 'reading a novel of Susan Hill's in which I failed to find a single semi-colon'. George Orwell, not usually dull of language, has been charged by Bernard Crick (1981, p. 254) with 'technical eccentricity' in deciding that his *Coming Up for Air* could manage without semicolons.

An opposite, more inventive, kind of eccentricity was used in James Baldwin's *Just Above My Head*, in which colons are used with novelty:

> I have been very frightened, for: I have had to try to strip myself naked.

> – it was largely because of Jimmy that Arthur became: a star: I do not mean . . .

Iris Murdoch interestingly and effectively used double punctuation in *The Sea, The Sea*:

> 'We shall all go with you, as a show of force, but also to back up your statement.'
> 'My statement?!'

Christine Brooke-Rose departed much further from the conventional mode in her novel *Thru*:

> Yes but they never went, that far, and you made me pay my God you did, and I always stopped when I saw, you were hurt, so I suffered both, the detach,ment and your, punishment, you'd go off for, days, and nights, whereas . . .

Another woman writer, Gertrude Stein, would presumably have found the excessive commas perverse. She even thought the comma was 'just a nuisance . . . If you think of a thing as a whole, and the comma keeps sticking out, it gets on your nerves: because, after all, it destroys the reality of the whole' (Stein, 1977, p. 153).

It has often been noticed that these eccentricities, reflecting personal peculiarities of intonation, have been more or less institutionalized by idiosyncrasies of speech style adopted by some broadcasters who use pauses and variations of stress and pitch to 'point up' words and phrases of special significance, e.g. when introducing a famous guest speaker. Crystal (1987b, p. 179) has reprinted an editorial in the *Guardian*, a newspaper notorious some years ago for its misprints. The writer demonstrates how odd broadcast 'mispronunciations' might look in print:

> The BBC has introduced a. New method of disseminating the spoken word at any rate we think it is new because we don't. Remember hearing it until a week or two ago

it consists of. Putting the fullstops in the middle of sentences instead of at the end as we were. Taught at school . . .

Such variations from normal usage are doubtless deviations exploited by professional writers perfectly conversant with ordinary practice. But teachers are necessarily concerned with unintended deviations from standard practice in non-literary language. Misuse of punctuation is often blamed for causing ambiguity. An employee is said to have lost her job because an intrusive comma turned her written accusation against a senior member of staff into an unintended resignation. She had written:

Mrs Pepperell is out to make my life hell, so I give in my notice.

(She meant that Mrs Pepperell tormented her *in order that* she, the writer, should leave.)

A more common potential ambiguity may occur when a negative is followed by 'because of', as in:

I'm not wearing my new hat because I don't like it.

(the hat was a present from her husband, but presumably unworn for other reasons) or

It would be unreasonable to debar them, because of inadequate staff.

or

She didn't marry him because of his religious beliefs.

In these cases – and in other syntactic constructions (for example, distinguishing between restrictive and descriptive clauses) – meticulous punctuation, either using or omitting a comma, in theory prevents ambiguity in writing; corresponding intonation patterns ought to do the same for spoken utterances. But in actual practice, unless (as often happens) a disambiguating context prevents misunderstanding, the presence or absence of a single comma can fail to carry the appropriate semantic load.

One of the more practical proposals for a change which would deal with the vexed problem of the possessive apostrophe, often and notoriously misused, is simply to abolish it. A headmaster in the 1960s (not, presumably, the 1960's!) wanted to form a Society for the Abolition of the Apostrophe. He maintained convincingly that that punctuation mark is not necessary, cannot be taught successfully to most users, and lends an appearance of illiteracy to otherwise accurately written work. We are all aware of the disappearance of the apostrophe from upper-case titles (such as LLOYDS BANK, DAME ALLANS BOYS SCHOOL), its intrusion where it is superfluous (as in Apple's for Sale; Coffee's, Grill's and Snack's; even, outside the Savoy Theatre some years ago, TAXI'S ONLY), and wrong placement (for example, childrens' mistakes; Keat's poetry). According to one scholar: 'After a brief period of relative stability during the late nineteenth and early twentieth centuries, the genitive apostrophe is gradually returning to the confusion from which it has recently emerged.' She regards it as 'a grammatical anomaly, a vestigial case-marker – appropriately shaped like the human appendix – in a noun system that has otherwise dispensed with cases' (Sklar, 1976–7, p. 175).

The small number of punctuation symbols available in English causes the same device – the 'crooked mark' or 'hook' – to be used both as a possessive and as an elision marker. Burchfield (1985, p. 25), with his usual sense of balance, deprecates the possible loss of the second type because it would produce 'Ill / shell / well / hell be seeing you', but thinks that the 'moderately useful' possessive device 'should be abandoned'. The muddled history of pronominal forms, for many years requiring possessive 'it's' as well as 'your's', 'our's' and so on, has led to clear precepts but not to more consistent practice. A recent 'junk-mail' leaflet advertised a 'genuine lead crystal goblet'. The picture of it was accompanied by messages which announced 'It's yours free' and assured you that 'your very own' goblet 'will be beautifully engraved with your family name and it's [*sic*] associated Coat-of-Arms.' Reviewing Burchfield's *The English Language*, Kingsley Amis declared (*Observer*, 28 January 1985) that abandoning the apostrophe would unloose 'a flood of ambiguity'. When challenged, he gave no examples of this dreaded ambiguity. In spite of the overwhelming evidence that human decisions about language-use have precious little effect on actual use (the living language being, as an American scholar observed, like a cowpath, created by cows themselves who follow it or depart from it according to their whim or their needs), Amis persists in pontificating. His rapid and complete failure, in alliance with John Wain and others, to resist the invasion of the sentence-adverbial use of 'hopefully' has apparently not discouraged him. Though language changes and – according to some observers – changes at an ever-increasing rate, punctuation remains and is likely to remain one of its most stable features, in Britain and probably wherever writing and printing systems dominate communication.

Stable syntax

This essential part of grammar concerns how words are put together to form structured sequences (phrases, clauses, sentences, discourses). Different languages use syntactic arrangements differently, but all languages – at least all well-known languages – seem to make basic structures that contain a noun-phrase subject (S), a verb or predicate (V), with sometimes a noun-phrase object or complement (O). The ordering of these three components varies. English, French, Spanish and Russian prefer the SVO order for statements. Japanese and Korean apparently prefer the SOV pattern. Classical Hebrew and Welsh, we are told, are VSO languages, but no languages have been discovered favouring the VOS order (see Fromkin and Rodman, 1978, p. 335). Utterances other than statements (questions, orders, exclamations) can ring the changes on these arrangements. So does 'poetic licence', as in the Milton lines quoted above (p. 49) and variations for the sake of particular emphasis (as in 'Talent, Mr Micawber has; capital, Mr Micawber hasn't'). But, whatever the range of basic patterns and of deviations from them, those patterns remain comparatively fixed and stable.

The forces ensuring syntactic stability include: the obvious need for a language to survive as an agent of thought, expression and communication; the powerful influence of recorded and retrievable written language; the conception of a standard language from which varieties can (but without which could not) diverge in accents and dialects, in creoles and pidgins, in stylistic usage (as in poetry and puns). However, stability does not mean permanent fixedness. Not only have attempts to 'fix' language proved futile, but a degree of change is essential for the sake of vitality. Lounsbury (1908, p. 7) makes the ironical point that 'in order to have a language become dead, it is first necessary that those who speak it should become dead – dead at least intellectually, if not physically'.

Whereas phonological, morphological and lexical changes have been well explored and charted, syntactic change has been less closely studied. One expert in the field – William Labov (1972, p. 65) – notes that 'Syntactic change is an *elusive* process as compared to sound change; whereas we find sound change *in progress* in every large city in the English speaking world, we have comparatively little data on syntactic change'(emphasis added). Presumably, the investigation of sound change has been greatly facilitated by sound-recording machines, but synchronic emphasis (*in progress*) draws attention to the slowness of syntactic change. It is probably too slow to be significantly recognized – even in written form – within a lifetime. Over centuries, changes in English syntax have been extensively documented with written quotation from Anglo-Saxon ('cume an spearþe and hrædlice, þæt hūs þurhflēo' meaning '(there should) come a sparrow and quick that house through-flies' – Strang (1970, p. 403) and from Shakespeare (for example, Prospero's 'Thy shape invisible retain thou still'). Neoclassical predilections thriving in the seventeenth and eighteenth centuries strove to restore to the English language regularities and rules emulating those derived from the dead classical languages.

Notorious prescriptions such as the prohibition of final prepositions (ostensibly because they should always be *pre*posed) and double negatives, condemnations of offences against case government in pronouns (between you and I) and concord (Everybody . . . their), confusion of usage (that/who/which) – these and many other such invented 'rules' persisted long enough to become the subject of record and advice in the Fowlers' *The King's English* (1906). In *Notes and Queries*, vehement armchair critics kept alive, at least into the twentieth century, issues about 'fused participles' ('Do you mind my/me smoking a cigar?'). The more ferocious pedants condemned the verb usage in, for example, 'The house is *being built*'. They rated this construction – which was to become standard – as an illiterate modification of 'The house is *building*', a construction which is, with few exceptions, now almost obsolete. A more recent defiance of change defended what was surely on the way to extinction; it is difficult even to remember what was at issue, namely, the alleged necessity of distinguishing 'up to' from 'down to' according to the relevant historical period. The 'rule' (or myth) that was invoked required a speaker or writer to use 'up to' for a date preceding historical records but 'down to' thereafter.

Though matters of English usage (including some of the items just mentioned) seem to fascinate the general public and to produce a multitude of anecdotes, as yet they have generated comparatively few sizeable language books. Mittins *et al.* (1970) examined variable judgements of fifty or so 'divided' usages. David Crystal (1984) asked – by means of his title – *Who Cares About English Usage?*, and Walter Nash (1986) offered a guide to first principles in his *English Usage*. The central problem posed by the fact that language remorselessly changes was specifically considered by Jean Aitchison (1981). She agrees with Labov that syntactic change is puzzling and elusive. She argues that de Saussure's separation of diachronic from synchronic linguistics and his contention that the opposition between these two points of view 'is absolute and allows of no compromise' (Aitchison, 1981, p. 125) discouraged investigation of language change. It remains true, of course – as Bloomfield had stated in 1933 and Hockett (1968, p. 85) had reaffirmed much later – that change cannot be directly observed as it happens; we can only detect it from its consequences. But, given the latitude of looking at language behaviour from a more detached position than the here and now – that is, at evidence supplied over at least a few generations and at variations in dialects, creoles and pidgins – some tentative generalizations become possible within a single language.

In these terms, we can ask: what changes in English syntax seem to be occurring? Aitchison (1981, p. 82) generously includes morphology as part of syntax; for her, syntactic change is 'change in the form and arrangement of words'. Even so, her examples are few. They include:

1 The often observed and long-established practice of 'conversion', that is, of converting one part of speech into another. She gives as examples 'Henry *downed* a pint of beer', 'Drusilla *garaged* her car', 'Bertie *upped* his score'. From non-standard teenage subculture she quotes '*chins* them with bottles' (hits on chin), 'We *bunks* it over here a lot' (play truant), and 'We *legs* it up Blagdon Hill' (run away). She could have mentioned many others, for example the popular new verb 'to rubbish'. There seems little doubt that the verbifying phenomenon is becoming increasingly noticeable.

2 An increase in the use of the progressive 'to be' form plus '-ing', not just for an action in progress (as in 'What are you reading?') but also for a matter of habitual behaviour ('Felix is tired of whisky; he'*s drinking* gin these days') or a mental state ('Charles *is understanding* French a lot better since he's been to Paris').

3 A decline in the frequency of impersonal verbs, dropping such constructions as 'It seems that . . .', 'It happens to be on Friday . . .'.

In Aitchison's view, some of these developments have the effect of simplifying, of tidying up, of 'neatening' the syntax. This 'neatening' process exemplifies 'the tendency to eliminate pointless variety' and 'a preference for constructions which are clear and straightforward' (Aitchison, 1981, p. 155). To that extent, they can be seen to strengthen the central stability of the syntactic patterns of English.

In general, while necessarily accepting what Sapir (1921, Ch. 7) aptly calls the 'drift' of language over centuries and recognizing that varieties of English and abuses of English often deviate from any 'standard' pattern – especially in the strict sense of ordering words – English syntax is very stable. Burchfield (1985, pp. 157–8) summarizes the situation as one in which 'No construction is everlastingly stable, no cherished rule remains unbroken' but 'At any given time it is safe to assume that permissible patterns of syntax are ascertainable if one has the means of identifying and classifying them'.

Versatile vocabulary

It is in lexis, the stock of words in a language, that change is most noticeable. The distinction (used in Chapter 4) between paradigmatic and syntagmatic words – in various terminologies referred to, on the one hand, as *lexical, vocabulary, content, open-class, full, contentive* words, and, on the other hand, as *grammar, function, closed-system, empty, functor* or *form* words – is not as clear-cut as is sometimes assumed. 'The first group [the paradigmatic ones] comprises the bulk of the lexicon of a language like English' (Carter and McCarthy, 1988, p. 206). The actual size of this group changes as new words are constantly, and apparently with increasing rapidity, added to it. Neologisms range from words made necessary by the needs of society to *hapax legomena* used only once. (Perhaps Mikes's 'eatard' – paralleling 'drunkard' – and Mencken's invention of 'ecdysiast' for 'stripper' qualify for the unique title.)

New words that are neologistic in form only, while increasing lexical resources, do not in themselves have a serious impact on stability or changeability. More significant are words that are semantically neologistic by adapting already familiar words to provide new meanings. The various semantic aspects of 'adapting' can be roughly classified as follows:

1 *Narrowing* has occurred, for example, to the extent that the generic term 'corn' usually denotes wheat in England, oats in Scotland, maize in America. Feminism has had some success in restricting 'man' (which did not connote gender) to 'male human being'. The traditional use of 'verbal', meaning *in words*, is giving way to a more limited sense equating it with 'oral'.
2 *Broadening*, which happens more frequently, has allowed 'literacy' to extend beyond competence specifically in writing and reading to cover spoken ability. Purists have failed to stop the verb 'to strand' being broadened to apply to men trapped in a submarine, or the noun 'ship' being extended to cover vehicles not water-borne (as in 'airship').
3 *Pejoration* happens when a word acquires a less favourable meaning than it previously had. This tendency is exemplified today by 'professional'. Hitherto

normally a term of approval, it has become associated with 'professional crimes' (e.g. by American White Supremacy thugs and by British 'professional fouls' in soccer). An older but better-known deterioration caused 'vulgar' to lose its neutral sense of 'popular' and connote something to be deplored.

4 *Melioration* has enabled 'enthusiasm', at one time strongly disapproved as meaning 'irrational' or 'frenzied', to become praiseworthy as connoting admirable qualities of energy and keenness. (Susie Tucker wrote a whole book (1972) about this particular 'shift'.) Similarly, 'sophisticated' has lost its etymological connexion with 'sophistry' and acquired an enviable sense of smartness or cleverness.

5 Changes of *substantive quality*, shifting meanings from concrete to abstract or vice versa, have deprived 'humour' of its physical sense (as in the four humours of medieval physiology) and made it refer normally to qualities of disposition marked by light-heartedness or amusement. Conversely, 'dedicated' is extending its concrete application to inscriptions and roadways and now to computers, with less common collocations with religious or moral devotion.

These and other vocabulary changes on the whole enlarge lexical resources, by contrast with Orwell's notorious Newspeak exercise (see above, p. 53), which sought – for pernicious political purposes – to prune vocabulary. The important question is whether movements in vocabulary make 'closeness of verbal fit' more possible or less attainable in a changing world. Since, irrespective of semantic change, there appear to be many more neologistic additions than word-meaning losses, the answer would seem to be at least that lexical resources are not decaying and at most that an increased vocabulary offers more lexical choices and therefore a greater possibility of close fit. The question of turning the potential into the actual is a pedagogical problem rather than a matter of assessing language stability or change.

7 Social variation

> *Scholer*: May I then never use my proper country termes, in writing?
> *Maister*: Yes: if they be peculiar termes, and not corrupting of words:
> As the Northren man writing to his privat neighbour may say: My
> *lathe* standeth neere the *kirke garth*, for My *barne* standeth neere
> the *Churchyard*. But if he should write publikely, it is fittest to use
> the most known words.
>
> (E. Coote, 1596)

Standard and non-standard varieties

The first three of Sinclair's (1985) 'six easy lessons' (pp. 25, 40 above) have
provided starting-points for our Chapters 4–6. These chapters have focused on
the nature of language – in turn, its productivity, its creativity, its stability. The
implication has been that teachers of language need to be aware of, and informed
about, issues raised by educational linguistics. The remaining three 'easy lessons'
shift the focus from the language *to be used* to the *uses* of language employed by
users. These matters invade the territory of sociolinguistics, pragmatics and
discourse analysis. For teachers the particular relevances involve, respectively,
social varieties of language, individual variations in language use, and conversation (in the broadest sense of language intercourse). Each of the areas of
sociolinguistics, pragmatics and discourse analysis is a sizeable academic discipline in its own right, generating specialist 'literatures' often occupying many
library shelves. Obviously, no single book on language awareness can be expected
usefully to cover all three fields. Moreover, a single writer cannot be expected to
do more than touch upon a few of the important aspects bearing most closely on
language teaching.

Under Sinclair's (1985) fourth title – 'social variation' – it is appropriate to start
from the notion of standard languages. One short working definition of a
standard language makes it 'a prestige variety of language used within a speech
community.' The definer adds that ' "Standard languages/dialects/varieties" cut
across regional differences, providing a unified means of communication, and
thus an institutionalized *norm* which can be used in the mass-media, in teaching
the language to foreigners, and so on' (Crystal, 1980, p. 329). In attempting to pin
down the highly complicated notion of a standard language, this short statement –
to some extent *because* it is short – makes arguable distinctions, raises contro-
versial issues, and introduces many variables. It is necessary to be aware of the
problem of distinguishing a dialect from a language, of mapping the many

varieties embraced by a single language, of grappling with the evaluative connotations of the terms 'standard', 'prestige', and 'norm'. But time and space do not permit of sorting out implications, much less of presenting an alternative terminology and 'model'. For our purposes, a standard language is a general-purpose language in common use in a speech community. Generously inter-preted, it is the language used in educational institutions, in much journalism, in communication by the mass media. It is also the chosen variety for foreign learners learning a second language. In other words, it can be negatively defined by what it is *not*, just as the total English language has been defined or at least circumscribed as any language that is not French, German, etc. By this method, Standard English (SE) is not substandard or non-standard language, it is not a medium for extremely colloquial conversation, it is not slang, it is not jargon used by an in-group of specialists, it is certainly not gobbledegook.

So long and so far as 'dialect' denoted one of many regional varieties making up a language, it was possible to say that a standard language was not a dialect. More recently, for democratic ideological reasons which insist (fairly) that all varieties are linguistically equal and none more equal than others, standard language has been 'equalized' as itself a dialect. There are, of course, many languages or dialects which can be called 'standard' according to one or more of a number of criteria – because they are 'national' or 'official' or 'educated' or because they offer 'norms' (for schools and colleges) or are 'internationally exportable' (in publications or broadcasts).

The HMI *English from 5 to 16*, also referred to as Curriculum Matters 1 (DES, 1984), provoked some adverse criticism by using the term 'Standard Spoken English'. Seeking, in *Responses to Curriculum Matters 1* (1986), to clarify the relevant issues, the Inspectorate quoted (in para. 30) a few sentences from an article by Peter Strevens (1985). The essential elements in Strevens's argument – accepted in the Kingman (DES 1988) and Cox (DES and Welsh Office, 1988b; 1989) reports – are:

> that 'Standard English has become the only acceptable model or target *for normal educational use*', that '"Standard English" really ought to be called the grammar and the core vocabulary of educated usage in English', and that Standard English dialect (remember we are referring to patterns of grammar and vocabulary and not to pronunciation) has no local base. On the contrary, it is accepted throughout the English-speaking world. And it is spoken with any accent. Consequently Standard English is the only dialect which is neither localised in its currency nor paired solely with its local accent.

Though SE is spoken as well as written, it is most typically recognizable in writing. Written and printed English, used, for instance, in official publications, in academic writing, in school textbooks and examination papers, exploits more of the vocabulary and syntax, which have incidentally been 'greatly elaborated' (DES and Welsh Office, 1988b, para. 5.45). This Report usefully summarizes the educational purposes of SE. It argues (para. 3.14) that SE should:

extend the range of varieties of English in which children are competent. From a developmental point of view this will mean adding to the local varieties used within the family and peer group those varieties used for wider communication (in school and higher education, in adult work and society): it means adding written language to spoken language, Standard English to non-Standard English, literary language to non-literary language (and, for children who have a different mother-tongue, adding English to their first language). It is clear that these extensions enable children to do more with their language. For example, they can do more when they can produce written language because they can write to people who are far away, or to institutions, government departments, newspapers etc; they can keep written records; they can write down ideas in order to reflect upon them and reformulate them; they can elaborate complex arguments which require written support; they can create and keep artistic artefacts – poems, plays, stories; and so on. They can do more when they have a mastery of Standard English because they can communicate in a wider circle both socially and geographically.

To insist – as many linguists do – on calling SE a dialect and on giving all dialects equal status is decently objective. It denies that being different in any way means being linguistically better or worse in serving its purpose. Nevertheless, popular usage still commonly accords social prestige or status to the standard variety. The same kind of upgrading occurs with American English. Fromkin and Rodman (1978, p. 258) offer a comparison with baseball:

> Even though every language is a composite of dialects, many people talk and think about a language as if it were a 'well-defined' fixed system with various dialects diverging from this norm. This is analogous to equating the American Baseball League of the 1950s to the New York Yankees. The Yankees enjoyed so much success in that decade that many baseball enthusiasts did just that. Similarly, a particular dialect of a language may enjoy such prestige that it becomes equated with the language itself.

Linguists recognize a Standard American English (SAE), calling it a standard dialect. As a norm – inevitably a theoretical, idealized norm – it distinguishes itself negatively by not being Philadelphia dialect, Boston dialect, Black English (BE), and so on. In the first edition of their book, Fromkin and Rodman (1974, p. 251) slip in neatly a snide remark that SAE is 'a dialect of English which many Americans *almost* speak'. This reminds one of Clarence Darrow's question: 'Even if you do learn to speak correct English, who are you going to talk it to?' Lyons (1981b, p. 270) suggests that 'it would be more reasonable to classify Australian English or Indian English under "British" than it is so to classify Scottish English and Irish English'. Logical categorizing might conceivably require SAE to be contrasted with Standard Canadian, Australian, South African, Jamaican, etc., English. The acronymic problem would be difficult enough without trying to classify Standard English English (of England) as distinct from Standard Scottish English and the 'Scots' language cherished by the Saltire Society. English-based pidgins and the creoles that grew from them are presumably too distant from any English 'norm' to claim, or indeed to want, recognition as in any sense forms of SE.

Some languages or dialects achieve their dominant status because, among other things, they are associated with capital cities of countries. Historically this was originally a factor in promoting the East Midland English dialect to become the standard English language. In France, the Parisian dialect is now regarded as the official French language and as such is protected by the Académie Française. In Italy, the eminence of Florence (the capital of Tuscany) seems to have assured the future of the Tuscan dialect as the official Italian language. A dominant dialect is, as we have said, normally the one chosen for the teaching of the relevant tongue as a second or foreign language. Most foreigners cannot be expected to master more than one variety of English, however intrigued they may be by regional dialects such as Geordie, Scouse, Cockney, etc. When Europeans, Asians, North Africans and even South Americans take refresher courses in England (such as those organized by the British Council), they expect and demand that these courses focus on Standard English English. Though they may be well travelled in the USA and certainly will recognize the numerical preponderance of speakers of American English in the West, they want – for themselves and, if they are teachers, for their students – Standard English as used in England. Arguments for favouring American English are from time to time put forward, as are arguments promoting the case for favouring non-standard British English in the teaching of English to native English-speakers. Nevertheless, it is an expert American phonologist who concedes that what Daniel Jones had described as Received Pronunciation (RP), that is, as 'universally accepted' pronunciation, characterizes this 'more fashionable accent' as 'the only dialect which continental Europeans and non-native speakers in the Commonwealth have thought worth speaking' (Kreidler, 1989, p. 294).

Registers

Dimensions of social variation have been dealt with under the name of 'institutional linguistics', which studies the relationships between types of situation and varieties of language. Much of the work in this area draws on the framework provided in *The Linguistic Sciences and Language Teaching* (Halliday *et al.*, 1964). In that book varieties of language are divided into two sets of sublanguages, dealing respectively with dialects and registers. One or two others have named the same distinction as between the dialectal and the diatypical. Though the name 'dialect' is well understood as the subject of the big discipline of dialectology or dialect geography, the term 'diatypical' has remained esoterically rare in use. 'Register', both as a label and as a concept, has also encountered some resistance. According to Crystal (1969, p. 307) 'only a minority of the world's linguists make use of the term (or even the concept) at all'. The objection to the word is presumably that it adds an extra and unnecessary meaning to an already polysemic term long used to refer to a written record, a recording apparatus (as in 'cash register') or a musical sound dimension (a range of vocal tone). This objection seems to have been outweighed by the term's usefulness (albeit *faute de mieux*) for linguists and teachers. The more serious substantive objection turns on complaints that the notion of register is unscientifically 'fuzzy'. It is totally dismissed in one book (O'Donnell and Todd, 1980, pp. 62–3), which rules that

> the register approach is spurious, and the notion is therefore ultimately unhelpful. In particular, the implication is to be strongly resisted that there exist discrete 'registers', or that the relationship between a given situation and the language occurring in that situation is ever close enough to enable us to identify a particular 'register'.

The authors find it 'misleading to imply that each situation may be objectively defined by reference to "parameters" such as field, tenor and mode' (Gregory and Carroll, 1978) and take the view that what they see as the vagueness and superficiality of most register discussions is probably caused by the unsatisfactory notion of register. Whether the study of language, that is, linguistics, should or could be objectively scientific in the modern strict sense remains disputable. If to take seriously notions of 'fuzzy' distinctions, of 'more or less' accurate analyses, of scalar clines, continua, gradability – all of these being familiar linguistic terms – is to be unscientific, so be it, because language itself is on these terms unscientific and the study of it necessarily less than rigorous.

One might claim that 'scientific' and 'unscientific' are themselves gradable terms. Their variable meanings extend from the strictly scientific (as, presumably, in the physical sciences) to a less absolute notion that includes degrees of probability not susceptible to exact measurement or demarcation. The comparatively new study of semantics none the less aims at a degree of precision. To that extent it can, as Leech (1969, p. 83) maintains, be distinguished from register:

> Semantics, like grammar and phonology, is a systemic study, concerned with all-or-none choices, whereas register is primarily a probabilistic study, concerned with the likelihood of one choice rather than another in a given type of social situation.

According to Halliday *et al.* (1964, p. 87) 'a dialect is a variety of language distinguished by the *user*', whereas a register is a variety 'according to *use*' (emphasis added). They proceed to make a threefold division of register into:

(a) field of discourse – broadly subject area, for example, politics, family affairs, law, religious practice, sports commentaries, auctioneers' 'patter';
(b) mode of discourse – broadly, speech or writing;
(c) style of discourse – determined by relationships between participants, and exemplified by the different styles adopted by a headmaster addressing colleagues, parents, schoolboys, caretakers, cleaners.

In the broader context of international English, the two sides of the distinction are less independent. The differentiation between American and British Englishes, for example, raises larger issues. Quirk (1989), supporting the Kingman

Committee's emphasis on standard English and resisting 'liberation linguistics', proposes an alternative taxonomy. Starting with *use*-related varieties as distinct from *user*-related varieties, he points out that, whereas it is not normal to switch between the two user-related varieties, two lawyers corresponding across the Atlantic both switch into 'legal English' (1989, p. 15).

Obviously, register is more or less independent of dialect. The fields, modes and styles can in principle be managed in any of the dialects available and communicatively suitable. In practice, dialectal features are much more notice-able in the spoken than in the written mode, and some fields of discourse (conspicuously for church or legal affairs) strongly favour the standard dialect and RP. Nevertheless, there are many markedly dialectal speakers (such as Lord Denning, John Arlott and a number of academic dons) who are prominent in public life.

The study of register has not yet produced an agreed terminology. The three sub-register categories have alternative names to those proposed by Halliday and his co-authors:

for field – 'province', 'domain'
for mode – 'medium', 'code'
for style – 'tenor', 'manner'.

The term 'register' is sometimes itself equated more narrowly with 'field' or 'code' or 'style'. Some scholars, while accepting 'register', have subclassified it along four instead of three dimensions, these being called 'field', 'mode', 'role' and 'formality'.

The twofold division of language varieties according to users (dialects) and use (registers) can be regarded as somewhat arbitrary and over-simple. In the words used by Halliday *et al.* (1964, p. 87), dialect users are 'different groups of *people* within the language community' and register is needed 'when we want to account for what *people* do with their language' (emphasis added). The simple words 'user' and 'use' are attractive, especially for teaching purposes, but the shared reference to 'people' tends to blur the distinction between personal characteristics (of place, schooling, social class, etc.) and personal language habits. Catford's (1965, pp. 84–90) analysis establishes a different twofold categorization into those which are more or less *permanent* for a given performer or group of performers; and those which are more or less *transient* in that they change with changes in the immediate situation of utterance. This distinction is the basis for Catford's more elaborate mapping of language varieties. The permanent characteristics include

idiolect: a particular individual's variety (for example, idiosyncratic pronuncia-tion or vocabulary)
dialect: a variety used by a group, often sharing features of space, time and social class

Transient features are related to the immediate situation of utterance. They include register: a variety correlated with social roles (for example, as, according to situation, head of family or motorist or cricketer or professor)

style: a variety identifiable along a scale roughly extending from formal to informal

mode: a variety of medium, basically spoken or written.

These characteristics can be further refined, modified and subdivided. The language of recognized literature might logically be regarded as a register in the Hallidayan theoretical framework, but it is more of a super-register; it bursts through most of the boundaries specified. Its 'field of discourse' is as infinitely extensive as human experience; its 'mode of discourse' is predominantly written or printed (as for libraries) but also spoken (as in storytelling, readings aloud, drama); its 'style of discourse' is all-inclusive of personal and social relationships. The dimension of 'mode' has yielded a complex chart recognizing variations within both speaking and writing (Figure 3). Gregory and Carroll (1978, pp. 38–47) explain and exemplify (a)–(h):

(a) conversing – spontaneous interchange between two or more people, possibly involving 'intimacy signals', 'silence fillers', 'sentence-sharing'
(b) monologuing – one individual, excluding possibility of interruption by others (for example, by crashing bores)
    – preachers, laywers, teachers, etc., speaking without scripts
(c) 'reciting' – telling stories, poems
(d) speaking of what is written to be spoken as if not written – speaking play texts
(e) speaking of what is written to be spoken – lectures, political speeches

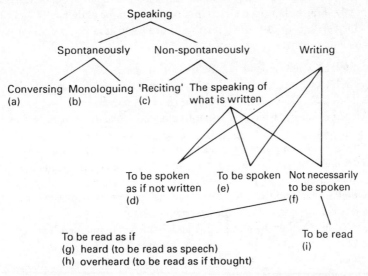

Figure 3 Varieties of mode
Adapted from Gregory and Carroll (1978, p. 47)

(f) speaking of what is written not necessarily to be spoken – telephone directories, novels
(g) speaking of what is written as if heard – actor performing, giving effect but not reality of spontaneous speech
(h) speaking of what is written to be read as if overheard – soliloquies

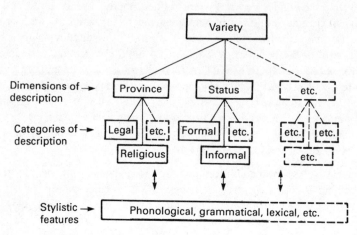

Figure 4   Statistical analysis
Derived from Allen and Corder (1973, p. 89)

Varieties of style have been mapped by Allen and Pit Corder (1973, p. 89), producing a different and more complex arrangement of dimensions and features (Figure 4). Those allergic to charts may prefer the same authors' list (p. 88) of 'at least thirteen sub-questions (referring to the English language) about what an utterance may answer':

Does it tell us which specific person used it? (*Individuality*)
Does it tell us where in this country he is from? (*Regional dialect*)
Does it tell us which social class he belongs to? (*Class dialect*)
Does it tell us during which period of English he spoke or wrote it, or how old he was? (*Time*)
Does it tell us whether he was speaking or writing? (*Discourse medium*)
Does it tell us whether he was speaking or writing as an end in itself or as a means to a further end? (*Simple versus complex discourse medium*)
Does it tell us whether there was only one participant in the utterance, or whether there was more than one? (*Discourse participation*)
Does it tell us whether the monologue and dialogue are independent, or are to be considered as part of a wider type of discourse? (*Simple versus complex discourse participation*)
Does it tell us which specific occupational activity the user is engaged in? (*Province*)

Does it tell us about the social relationship existing between the user and his interlocutors? (*Status*)

Does it tell us about the purpose he had in mind when conveying the message? (*Modality*)

Does it tell us that the user was being deliberately idiosyncratic? (*Singularity*)

Does it tell us none of these things? (*Common-core*)

Styles and situations

Stylistic features of register on a formal–informal scale have produced the set of levels or degrees exemplified by Martin Joos in his well-known *The Five Clocks* (1962). He compares the range of styles with the different hours recorded on clocks in the five time-zones extending across North America. Using much the same analogy, Fishman tells how

> A traveler in a foreign land once came to a five-sided clock tower. He walked round the tower and noticed that the clock on each side showed a different time. He stopped a native of the community and asked, 'Why do you need all of these clocks; they don't even show the same time?' 'That's exactly why we need them all,' he was told; 'If they all showed the *same* time, we could get along with just one!' (Fishman, in Miller, 1973, p. 274)

The moral is that we need a number of language varieties to match the range of situations in which we communicate.

Joos labelled and exemplified his 'five clocks' as:

Frozen: Visitors should make their way at once to the upper floor by way of the staircase.

Formal: Visitors should go up the stairs at once.

Consultative: Would you mind going upstairs, right away, please.

Casual: Time you all went upstairs, now.

Intimate: Up you go, chaps!

Strevens (1977, p. 145) quotes a set of examples giving essentially the same message but involving a wider range of situations and a variety of speakers, places and styles:

Frozen (e.g., over a public-address system) 'The lady in the back row wearing a fur coat is requested to keep silent.'

Formal (e.g., lecturer to known student) 'Be so good as to stop talking, Miss Jones.'

Consultative (e.g., at a small meeting with colleagues) 'Do you mind not talking at the moment, Miss Jones.'

Casual (e.g., at a meeting of friends engaged in discussion) 'Let's have quiet for a moment, please, Betty.'

Intimate (e.g., between two lovers in back row) 'Darling – shshsh!'

One writer (Rosaline Chiu) has equated these five styles with five corresponding social attitudes: hectoring, imperative, polite, ingratiating, wheedling. Other verbal labels have been preferred to those used by Joos. The terminology used by Graustein *et al.* in their *English Grammar* calls them in order stilted, formal, neutral, colloquial, intimate. Strevens (1965, p. 85) has urged that 'the analysis must take into account the feature of *vulgarity*', adding to Joos's five levels a sixth to accommodate vulgarisms such as 'Get up them stairs!' Graustein *et al.* intensified coarseness with 'Get up them bloody stairs!'

Whereas vulgarisms clearly belong to the bottom end of the scale, euphemisms graduate towards the frozen or formal end. English is rich in near-synonyms distinguished by appropriateness to various grades of register. Examples denoting common aspects of behaviour can accordingly be graded. It has often been pointed out, for example, that 'to die' falls between 'to kick the bucket' or 'to snuff it' (intimate or casual) and 'to expire' (consultative or neutral). Similarly, 'sexual intercourse' separates 'perform coitus with' from 'screw' and many other monosyllabic vulgarisms. A 'toady' or 'yes-man' may, at the extremes, be a 'sycophant' or an 'arse-licker' (Cruse, 1986, p. 285). Mixtures of register are as common as mixed metaphors. Presumably Gladstone spoke in an excessively formal style that led Queen Victoria to complain: 'He speaks to Me as if I was a public meeting.' Orwell was describing an obsolescent feature of educated register when, in *The Clergyman's Daughter*, he made the Rector deplore Dorothy's way of naming their midday meal:

> 'Luncheon, Dorothy, luncheon!' said the Rector with a touch of irritation. 'I do wish you would drop that abominable lower-class habit of calling the midday meal *dinner*!'

Awareness of language varieties and competence to use them are recognized to some extent by language teachers, but perhaps not to the extent recommended by Halliday (1978, p. 28), who argued that 'the ability to control the varieties of one's language that are appropriate to different uses is one of the cornerstones of linguistic success, not least for the school pupil'. Teachers and examiners also need to control registers carefully. A striking example of confusing registers has been quoted by Maureen Mobley in relation to 'readability in the GCSE'. To test students about the concept of viscosity, a question was asked about the problems of transporting oil across Alaska. Some candidates, particularly girls, associated Alaska with heat because 'baked Alaska' is a dessert sweet experienced perhaps in domestic science lessons, whereas 'Alaska', in the register of geography, connotes coldness. Similarly, and more seriously for candidates from 'ethnic' backgrounds, a question expressed in bleak examination language (itself a formidable register) presented: 'Sugar is a mixed blessing. Discuss.' This challenge produced answers that assumed that 'mixed blessing' was a pudding, rather like angel delight! (Working Paper No. 5, Secondary Examinations Council, 1987, p. 5).

That older and abler students do not always master the delicacies of appropriate register is revealed by a candidate for university entrance who, responding to a request to write a letter to a friend suggesting a part of England for a holiday visit, recommended camping in the Lake District. The writer used a mixture of the registers of geography, geology and travel agency salesmanship rather than a more personal, friendly style:

> The Lake District is a beautiful area, where majestic mountains rise into the overlying blanket [!] of clouds and the large mirror-like lakes sparkle where the rays of the sun penetrate the surface of the lakes. The area consists of undulating relief . . .
>
> The geomorphological features are fantastic in shape and size and these are a result of glacial action . . . There are a few depositional features to be seen, especially at Lake Windermere where it has been dammed by morraine . . .

Potential examiners might be invited to consider how seriously to penalize this lapse in a piece otherwise fairly competent in syntax and vocabulary.

An English language course aiming at reducing the occurrence of such offences might include, for example, exercises in:

1 Placing on the Joos scale utterances such as 'I think I'll get a bit of shut-eye' or (in a context of appointing a new colleague) ''Fraid you've picked a lemon.'
2 Upgrading an utterance along the Joos scale, e.g., providing the *formal* equivalent of 'Jaez, boss, get a load of dis'.
3 Inventing a twentieth-century utterance to rival the incident in which hot tea was spilled over the precocious young John Stuart Mill at a reception organized by his philosopher father for distinguished guests. When the offending visitor anxiously enquired whether John Stuart had been scalded, the youth is said to have replied: 'Madam, the anguish has somewhat abated.'
4 Identifying the nursery rhyme in:

   > Scintillate, scintillate, globule lucific.
   > Fain would I fathom thy nature specific.

5 Emulating the fictitious professor-cum-journalist who (in *The Times Higher Educational Supplement*) introduced a university debate with:

   > In the Blue corner – from the physics department – top of the lecturer's scale for nine years, I give you – Doctor Lionel Benskin. (Loud cheers) And in the Red corner . . .

6 Explaining the oddity about the barrister who impatiently called out to his wife: 'Come on, darling, hurry up. I will brook no delay' or the young man who said: 'It was extremely gracious of you to invite me, Lady Jones, and I've had lots of fun.'
7 Adding to a list of words (made up by Bolinger) expressing the same notion in Joos's categorization (intimate, casual, consultative, formal, frozen):

   > to guzzle, to swig, to drink, to imbibe, to quaff
   > nutty, crazy, insane, demented, mad.

It seems likely that – by any definitions of language and dialect – English, being increasingly a world language (cf. p. 15), has more varieties than most other languages. The catalogue of recognizable English registers is extensive enough to include a register which may be unique. Strevens (1965, pp. 83–4) suggests that, 'to the utter amazement of most foreigners', English people reserve a special spoken register 'for speaking to babies and small domesticated animals'.

Teachers of foreign languages are often so fluent that they extend their expertise into non-standard varieties of those languages. They may even achieve the distinction – often the criterion for judging native-like command of a language – of being able to swear in those languages. Learners of a foreign language, that is, those with whom we are for the moment primarily concerned, may in due course become fluent enough to be introduced to social variations (not necessarily for swearing!) relevant to problems of translating dialectal and register-specific utterances. But, in the main, mastery of the standard variety of a language remains the central objective in schools and in further education. There, familiarity with non-standard locutions will for some years develop only incidentally, normally from the registers used in common situations encountered in family life, in advertising and in popular journalism. These sources may be supplemented by the loan words and loan phrases (not usually included in core or nuclear vocabularies) that proliferate increasingly in serious journalism and in literature. The native-English reader is often assumed to understand 'déjà vu', 'esprit d'escalier', 'kindergarten', 'flak', 'ravioli', 'crescendo', 'sputnik', 'xenophobia', 'in flagrante delicto', 'mutatis mutandis', etc. (cf. p. 36).

8 How to do things with language – pragmatics

Varro [second century BC] illustrates the essentially pragmatic nature of language; speech was used for the daily needs of living long before it was treated as a means for the expression of systematized thought, and as Varro saw, those who look in language for a logically self-consistent and complete system are stressing a secondary and relatively recent function of language.

(R. H. Robins)

Indeterminacy

In the fifth of his 'Six Easy Lessons', Sinclair takes as theme – in his words – 'how to get things done, using language, while being aware that it may not be interpreted in exactly the way in which it is intended.' The gap between intention and interpretation is caused by the approximate, 'more or less' nature of language – its indeterminacy. A theoretical scale for measuring degrees of adequacy, of success in finding words to match meanings, would extend from maximal to minimal 'closeness of verbal fit'. At the maximum end would be, for example, an instruction (as in a test paper) to 'Multiply four by five and divide the result by two'. Our conventional decimal system seems to ensure totally meaningful clarity within that tautological system, but the message is very simple and barely verbal at all; it could be conveyed by non-verbal symbols: $(4 \times 5) \div 2 = $. (We note in passing, but dare not dwell on it, that even simple arithmetic supposedly gives less than total certainty. Whitehead (1948, p. 156) concedes that the proposition that 'Twice three is six' looks utterly certain, but he questions the absolute reliability even of that. Cardinal numbers, he says, are 'a battleground of controversy', because they rely on the concept of a class and the notion of a class is 'beset with ambiguities leading to logical traps'. Logic may be the 'chosen resort of clear-headed people' but, unfortunately, logicians cannot agree with each other!) Equally close to total communication of meaning are exchanges about very familiar things between pairs well known to each other (such as husband and wife or two old friends). But again words may play comparatively little part, being partially replaced by 'intimacy signals' (such as 'y' know', 'ah-ha', or even grunted noises).

More conventional and more 'public' utterances are much more susceptible to misunderstanding, ambiguity and incomprehensibility. A recent blatant example seems to have been experienced at considerable personal expense by a junior minister at the Ministry of Health. In a broadcast by ITN on 3 December 1988, she stated:

> We do warn people *now* that most of the egg production of this country, *sadly*, is *now* infected with salmonella. If, however, they have used a good source of eggs, a good shop that they know, and they are content, then there seems no reason for them to stop. But we would *advise strongly* against using raw egg – mayonnaise and dressing and Bloody Marys and that sort of thing. They are not a good idea any more. [my italics]

The alarm caused by this statement was such as to cause the House of Commons' Agriculture Committee to discuss what exactly was meant. The Minister's statement was printed and she was invited to explain. Her answer (in a letter dated 25 January 1989) was that:

> I did *not* mean and did not say, as was incorrectly reported in the Press, that most of the eggs in this country are infected. I intended to explain that a significant number of the egg-laying hens in many of the egg-laying flocks in this country are infected with salmonella . . .
> The contents of intact hens' eggs from flocks in England and Wales and abroad have been shown to be infected with the same type of salmonella [i.e. *S. enteridis* PT4]. [her emphasis]

The principal misunderstanding arose from the indeterminate phrase 'egg production'. In the event, the Minister replaced her reference to the process of 'production' (a somewhat vague, abstract concept) with more easily understood references to the physical process of 'egg-laying' and the very real product of actual 'eggs'. It became clearer that salmonella is a persistent infection that we humans have long lived with and can continue to live with. Mrs Currie's use of 'warn', especially associated with 'now' and 'not a good idea any more', not surprisingly, caused considerable alarm.

The unfortunate or ill-advised speaker might now share with Whitehead (1948, p. 73) the judgement that 'there is not a sentence which adequately states its own meaning'. This places single sentences at the minimum end of our adequacy scale. Teachers and lecturers in their role as examiners have often encountered the difficulty of so wording short questions that they do not elicit answers to alternative, unintended questions ('Splendid, but that's not what I asked!'). They, too, will be inclined to accept Whitehead's dictum. It may be that longer phrasing of questions – several sentences or a paragraph – would reduce misunderstanding. The Goodmans (1988, pp. 168–9), for instance, claim to have learnt through miscue analysis that 'other things being equal, short language sequences are harder to comprehend than long ones. Sentences are easier than words, paragraphs easier than sentences, pages easier than paragraphs, and stories easier than pages'. On the other hand, especially with 'loose' language, the more words and sentences, the more risks of accidental or deliberate misunderstanding.

In general, we must accept that maximum 'closeness of verbal fit' is unlikely except for trivial utterances or for expressions relying on non- or quasi-verbal symbols such as those which serve formal logic (for example $\sim$ and $\equiv$) and mathematics ($+$ and $\times$) or those which supplement speech with body language, gesture and facial expressions, that is, with kinesic features. (Teachers often have opportunities in drama lessons to encourage precision in communicating meaning through physical symbols.) In between the extremes we should obviously aim at an *optimum* level achieving whatever degree of clarity is appropriate to the relevant context.

The notion of complete precision in language use is mythical, a will-o'-the-wisp or *ignis fatuus* too often regarded reverently as (mixing our metaphors) a 'holy cow'. Many thinkers about language have in their various ways commented on this 'fict'. Russell (1948, p. 163), for example, argues that:

> Outside logic and pure mathematics [both relying on non-verbal symbols], there are no words of which the meaning is precise, not even such words as 'centimetre' and 'second'. Therefore, even when a belief is expressed in words having the greatest degree of which empirical words are capable, the question as to what it is that is believed is still more or less vague.

Widdowson (1983, p. 163) maintains that 'communication is always relative to purpose. It is never precise but is always approximate'. He endorses Popper's (1976, p. 24) contention that 'the idea of a precise language, or of precision in language, seems to be altogether misconceived ... *The quest for precision is analogous to the quest for certainty* [cf. p. 57 above] and both should be abandoned'. In their book about metaphors, Lakoff and Johnson (1980, pp. 231–2) conclude:

> When the chips are down, meaning is negotiated; you slowly figure out what you have in common, what it is safe to talk about, how you can communicate unshared experience or create a shared vision. With enough flexibility in bending your world view and with luck and skill and charity, you may achieve some mutual understanding.

The familiar idea that reading essentially involves guessing is echoed in Leech's (1983, p. 30) remark that 'interpreting an utterance is ultimately a matter of guesswork, or (to use a more dignified term) hypothesis formation'. If all these quotations look like a counsel of despair, we can at least stop short of sharing Gertrude Stein's wordily convoluted pessimism:

> Clarity is of no importance because nobody listens and nobody knows what you mean no matter what you mean, nor how clearly you mean what you mean. But if you have vitality enough of knowing enough of what you mean, somebody and sometime and sometimes a great many will have to realize that you know what you know what you mean and so they will agree that you mean what you know, what you know you mean, which is as near as anybody can come to understanding anyone. (1931/75, p. xxv)

Distinctions, classifications, systems

The academic study of language, faced with an intricate complex of phenomena, has naturally tried to reduce the total chaotic jumble to order. To this end, linguists have divided language into component systems, models and levels. They have devised diagrams to present these divisions. Morris (p. 29 above) identified 'three essential features of the prevailing classification'. He asserted:

A language is completely described in terms of the signification of its simple and compound signs, the restrictions which are imposed on sign combinations, and the way the language operates in the behavior of its interpreters. These distinctions are those of semantics, syntactics, and pragmatics.

The three components had been anticipated by the well-known 'triangle of reference' of Ogden and Richards. They emphasized that, while thought and reference are each linked directly with both a symbol and a referent, there is only an indirect, imputed connexion between the last two (Figure 5).

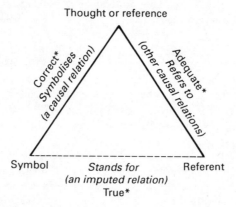

Figure 5   Semiotic triangle (a)
Derived from Ogden and Richards (1923, p. 11)

It has been remarked that Robert Browning anticipated the essence of the semantic triangle in a sentence in *The Ring and the Book*:

Art may tell a truth
Obliquely, do the thing shall breed the thought,
Nor wrong the thought, missing the mediate word.
(Book XII, lines 859–61)

Using Morris's more technical terminology and also replacing 'Thought or reference' with 'Interpreters', and 'Symbol' with 'Sign', Meredith (1956) developed a more elaborate semiotic triangle (Figure 6). The base-line here joining 'Signs' to 'Referents' might reasonably have been broken or dotted – as it is in the

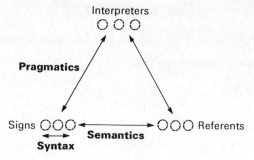

Figure 6   Semiotic triangle (b)
Derived from Meredith (1956)

Ogden–Richards diagram – to emphasize the merely imputed connexion between signs and the phenomena they denote. This would have reinforced the rejection of the persistent fallacy that meaning inheres *directly* in words.

Pragmatics

For educational purposes, language has recently been presented again as a compartmented set. The Kingman Report (DES, 1988; see Chapter 1 above) offers a 'model', not in the shape of a triangle, but as a set of linked 'boxes'. These, like other diagrammatic arrangements, are normally and necessarily accompanied by warnings against oversimplification. (Perhaps a multidimensional 'pop-up' device – such as, it is said, the Kingman Committee would have preferred to the fold-out arrangement actually used – would have needed less of a warning.) The distinctions made (for example, between syntax and semantics, between form and meaning) are relative rather than clear-cut; the categories used overlap and overflow into each other. The underlying process of classification itself is essentially *ad hoc*; it depends on which criteria are chosen to justify a differentiation. Bar-Hillel (1956, pp. 287–8) gives a parody of classification derived from mixed criteria. He fictitiously claims to have found six different ways of classifying fish:

1 edible – inedible
2 Mediterranean – other
3 over 3 inches long – 3 inches long or smaller
4 those whose species' name starts with *A* . . . with *B*, etc.
5 those which eat other fish but are eaten by no other fish – those which are eaten by other fish but eat no other fish – those which do both – those which do neither
6 blimpsy – blumpsy – bloompsy

Checking the impulse to ask which of these classifications was the correct one, he investigated their backgrounds:

And then I found that the men who proffered classification No.

1 was an economist
2 was an Italian
3 was the famous Eddingtonian fisherman
4 was a lexicographer
5 was an ecologist
6 was a philosopher who claimed that his classification was 'the only correct one on intuitive self-evident grounds'.

The moral of this story is: beware cross-classifications; they may express vested interests.

The title of this chapter – 'How To Do Things with Language' – takes us into the domain of pragmatics, which is concerned with the principles of *using* language. Bruner's view, shared increasingly by educationists, is that 'the route into language and learning and language and imbeddedness into society is pragmatics' (Bruner, 1975, p. 81). Traditionally (as noted in Chapter 2 above) the study of language has usually started with syntax before systematically considering semantics. The last thirty years or so have added pragmatics. Broadly speaking, and as far as possible avoiding the more technical terminology, the Kingman Report (DES, 1988) roughly follows this sequence. It seems sensible, as it has always seemed sensible, to start with relatively well-known and clear-cut matters of language forms before tackling more complex and less clear matters of language use. This order puts the purely linguistic before the sociolinguistic, which treats language as embedded in social contexts where meanings depend on extra-linguistic circumstances. It also gives priority to Saussure's *langue* over his *parole*, distinguishing the potential, abstract, ideal conception of language from actual verbal use. The former – *langue* – has been described as 'a system of mutually defining entities connected only arbitrarily with the reality of a string of utterances' (Lott, 1988, p. 3). Pragmatics deals less with 'entities' than with relationships.

Theoretical linguistics focuses on 'competence' rather than 'performance'. In the Chomskyan sense (as distinct from the ordinary everyday sense), linguistic 'competence' is knowing the rules of the game, frequently invoking chess as an analogue of the language-game. Educational linguistics, the sort of linguistics which can usefully act as a background for a teacher's knowledge of language (though not as material for direct teaching) concentrates more on 'performance', on how well the language game is played. Performance is analysed in pragmatics and, as Leech (1983, p. 35) says, 'must be concerned, quite centrally, with indeterminacy'. Though the academic study of pragmatics necessarily treats its subject more or less progressively as one of the various systems (others being systems of syntax, semantics, phonology, discourse), these dimensions are better regarded as a network than as a set of levels or layers – just as language as a whole is better regarded as an organism than as a machine. One writer, actually of a book on *Second Language Grammar*, remarks that deceptively facile terms (he specifically mentions 'code') are used for 'an unfathomably complex labyrinth of intertwining, overlaying, and convoluted phonological, syntactic, semantic, and pragmatic relationships' and that 'we may well wonder how the learner of another language manages to make any headway at all' (Rutherford, 1987, p. 7). We might even wonder how *any* language, including our native first one, is acquired – except that we are surrounded by overwhelming evidence that we all somehow make at least one language work.

Making it work still remains at a considerable distance from the comparatively recent emergence of theories of pragmatics. For our purposes it is advisable to pass quickly over systematic explication of principles and consider as much as possible samples of actual practice in communication. Since using language is, as the above quotation from Rutherford suggests, a kind of problem-solving exercise, it is reasonable to accept the approach used by Leech (1983). For him, the treatment of communication as problem-solving raises two basic problems, directed respectively at speakers and hearers:

> A speaker, *qua* communicator, has to solve the problem: 'Given that I want to bring about such-and-such a result in the hearer's consciousness, what is the best way to accomplish this aim by using language?' For the hearer, there is another kind of problem to solve: 'Given that the speaker said such-and-such, what did the speaker mean me to understand by that?' (Leech, 1983, p. x).

The considerations involved in communication are organized by Leech into categories of rhetoric which are in turn divided into principles and then into maxims. A fairly elaborate, not to say formidable, diagram charts these features as shown in Figure 7. In working through this programme, the author deals with

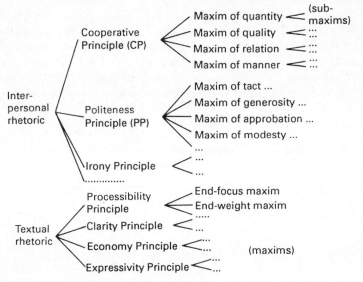

Figure 7   Communication as problem-solving
Derived from Leech (1983)

implicatures and entailments, with speech-act theory, and with many other matters relevant to linguists seeking to provide comprehensive descriptions of 'the things that one can do with words'. He also deals with matters less specifically related to pragmatics and already the concern of some teachers – such as discourse, irony, ambiguity, *oratio obliqua*, hyperbole, litotes. The language awareness of teachers could be enhanced both by extending these latter fairly familiar items and by accepting the relevance (more or less) of the 'pragmatics-specific' items mentioned.

Leech's use of 'rhetoric' approximates less to the traditional literary and public-persuading senses than to the educational sense in which it has been employed in America and in Scottish terminology (for example, in Grierson's textbook on *Rhetoric and English Composition*). In other words, it treats of 'the effective use of language in its most general sense, applying it primarily to everyday conversation, and only secondarily to more prepared and public uses of language' (Leech, 1983, p. 15). The binary division between textual and interpersonal rhetorics matches the division between the language-specific and the culture-specific extremes – the grammatical and the sociological ends – of his diagrammatic representation of general pragmatics (Figure 8).

Halliday has used the textual/interpersonal terminology in defining two of the three functions of language. In Leech's (1983, p. 56) words, Halliday's 'textual' was that of 'language functioning as a means of constructing a text', while the 'interpersonal' was that of 'language functioning as an expression of one's attitudes and an influence upon the attitudes and behaviour of the hearer'. (The third function – the ideational – was that of 'language functioning as a means of conveying and interpreting experience of the world'.) Central to these first two functions is the distinction between semantic 'sense' and pragmatic 'force', generated by the philosopher, J. L. Austin, in his speech-act theory. We can approach this via Leech's (1983, p. 195) ironic remark that 'the classification of illocutionary acts has been an important pastime of those wishing to make a thorough survey of "the things one can do with words"'. He is alluding, of course, to Austin's (1962) innovatory book on *How to do Things with Words*, which

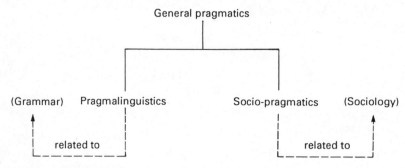

Figure 8 Pragmatic distinctions
Derived from Leech (1983, p. 11)

reprinted his William James lectures at Harvard University in 1955 and which expressed views formed even earlier, in 1939.

Speech-act theory

Exploring his notion of 'illocutionary force', Austin tentatively divided illocutionary acts or functions (he suggested there were 10,000 of them) into 'five very general classes'. He was 'far from equally happy about all of them' but gave them what he admitted were 'more-or-less rebarbative names'. Certainly they belied the engaging simplicity of what became the title of his book. He called them:

1 verdictives
2 exercitives
3 commissives
4 behabitives   ('a shocker this', he admitted)
5 expositives.

Austin proceeded to list five sets of verbs under these headings. Other scholars (for example, Wardhaugh, 1986; Flowerden, 1988) have developed the categorization with descriptions and examples, producing:

1 verdictives (e.g., estimate) – giving a verdict (as in 'We find them guilty')
2 exercitives (e.g., appoint) – exercising power or right (as in 'I pronounce you husband and wife')
3 commissives (e.g., promise) – promising or otherwise undertaking (as in 'I hereby bequeath')
4 behabitives (attitudes and social behaviour) – apologizing, congratulating (as in 'I'm sorry')
5 expositives (clarifying reasons, arguments . . .) – replying, arguing, conceding (as in 'I argue', 'I assume').

It is neither necessary nor obviously useful for teachers *qua* teachers to pursue pragmatics to this analytic extent or to use its rather disagreeable nomenclature, but it is desirable that they be aware of the general class of illocutionary speech acts. These are so called 'performatives' because they each perform an act *in saying* something; typically they are or could be marked – as the commissive example above is marked – with the adverb 'hereby' ('I *hereby* promise, appoint, name . . .'). This distinguishes them from locutions and perlocutions. Leech (1983, p. 199) contrasts

(a) an ordinary locutionary act, in which someone performs the act *of* saying something to somebody, with
(b) an illocutionary act, in which – as stated above – someone performs an act *in* saying something to somebody, and with
(c) a perlocutionary act, in which somebody performs an act *by* saying something to somebody.

In (a) a speaker says to a hearer that . . . ; in (b) the speaker asserts that . . . ; in (c) the speaker convinces a hearer that. . . .

Austin (1962, pp. 101–2) gives as examples:

Act (A) or	Locution
	He said to me 'Shoot her!' meaning by 'shoot' *shoot* and referring by 'her' to *her*.
Act (B) or	Illocution
	He urged (or advised, ordered, etc.) me to shoot her.
Act (C(a)) or	Perlocution
	He persuaded me to shoot her.
Act (C(b))	He got me to (or made me, etc.) shoot her.

For teaching purposes, this categorization involves Austin's (1962, p. 73) valuable distinction (mentioned above) between two aspects of meaning, between the ordinary *sense/reference* of an utterance which more or less literally transmits a message of factual information, and its *force*, which indicates 'how it is to be taken'. Distinctions such as this are ultimately indeterminate and fuzzy, but less so than the unsatisfactory traditional distinction merely between statements, questions and commands. This triadic differentiation is over-simple. It leaves out of account many of the uses of language, for example, its interpersonal function in reflection (self-communicating in sub-vocal thinking) and self-expression, its social function in 'phatic communion' as a social regulator promoting human warmth without sending an explicitly meaningful verbal message, its ceremonial and ritual purposes (as in religious services, in the chanting of protest or mass (dis)approval, and even in the child's use of 'kerb drill' as an incantation for warding off evil motor-cars). It overemphasizes transactional and informational purposes and underemphasizes expressive and poetic purposes, thereby casting users, especially learners, as – in Britton's terminology – 'participants more often than spectators'.

The other significant weakness of the statement/question/command simplification is in its blurring of form and function. Linguistic forms do not simply match communicative functions. Leech quotes as epigraph lines from Arthur Guiterman's *A Poet's Proverbs* in illustration of this:

Don't tell your friends about your indigestion;
'How are you!' is a greeting, not a question.

In fact, that exclamatory greeting has at least three possible meanings with three different intonation patterns:

1 'How *are* you!' could express surprise, both at the unexpectedness of meeting an old friend and at his remarkably healthy appearance (perhaps after an illness).
2 'How *are* you?' could be a doctor's genuine enquiry about how a patient feels.
3 'Good morning. How-er you' could be phatic – a perfunctory mutter prefacing

a serious business talk between strangers (for example, between a sales representative and a store's 'buyer').

Wilkins (1972, p. 147) points out that imperative forms are used for many purposes that are not conventionally imperative in the sense of giving orders. He lists:

Find a seat and I'll get the drinks	(suggestion)
Do that and I'll knock your teeth in	(threat)
Connect the hose to the water supply	(instruction)
Turn left at the traffic lights and take the third turning on the left	(direction)
Watch your glass	(warning)
Have a drink	(invitation)

Widdowson (1979, pp. 14–15) similarly shows how the 'imperative mood' construction is not restricted to 'commands' as traditionally understood. It can extend to serve an instruction ('Bake the pie in a slow oven'), an invitation ('Come for dinner tomorrow'), a prayer ('Forgive us our trespasses') or advice 'Take up his offer' (the last being equivalent to 'I should take up his offer').

Because of the nature of their work, teachers could conversely supply utterances which function as orders without containing any imperative forms. An injunction to be quiet (equivalent to 'Stop talking!') is often obliquely transmitted in the form of a statement ('Someone in the back row is talking') or a question ('Is it necessary for you to discuss the topic with your neighbour?'). School children learn quickly to appreciate the intended or 'real' meaning in spite of the surface forms of teachers' illocutions. In this, presumably because of the restricted contexts of school conditions and the limited co-texts of the curriculum, they do better than some adults in more complex and subtle situations. Better, for example, than the pair in Milan Kundera's *The Unbearable Lightness of Being*:

> he listened eagerly to the story of her life and she was equally eager to hear the story of his, but although they had a clear understanding of the logical meaning of the words they exchanged, they failed to hear the semantic susurrus of the river flowing through them.

Though a 'semantic susurrus' is pre-eminently a literary quality, it is paralleled in non-literary ordinary language by undercurrents of meaning often finding covert oblique expression. Leech seems to link this feature with *oratio obliqua*, a mode which, as indirect or reported speech, used to figure regularly and in a somewhat primitive way in composition exercises in schools and in public examinations. He argues that 'a performative is metalinguistic: it is, both syntactically and semantically, a kind of reported speech (*oratio obliqua*) utterance' (Leech, 1983, p. 181). Without either seeking to reinstate the now discredited mechanical school exercise or entering the abstrusely technical territory of 'pragmalinguistics', it is relevant briefly to consider obliqueness in communication. The commonest oblique utterances are probably those that employ irony. Leech's (1983, pp. 142–3) examples include 'That's all I wanted' (ironic exaggeration), Mark Twain's 'Some of his words were not Sunday school words' (ironic understatement) and ironic contradictions such as 'With friends like him, who needs enemies' and 'Bill wanted that news like he wanted a hole in the head!' Similarly, the strategy of hyperbole overstates (as in 'It made my blood boil'), while litotes or meiosis understates ('I wasn't overimpressed by her speech'). Lakoff, arguing that 'semantics cannot be taken to be independent of pragmatics, but that the two are inextricably tied together', pointed out that truth can turn on connotative meaning (often assumed to be 'the wastebasket of meaning') rather than literal meaning. His examples (Lakoff 1975, pp. 236–7) include the ironical use of 'regular', as in 'Esther Williams is a *regular* fish' (literally untrue) and 'John is a *regular* bachelor' (only said when he isn't a bachelor). Similarly, irony can offer highly dramatic examples of what Grice called 'conversational implicatures' (1981, pp. 183–98), as when a speaker (described in Miller and Johnson-Laird, 1976, p. 168) refers to someone he detests by saying 'Isn't he a great guy', meaning exactly the opposite.

The use of ironical language is a sadly neglected area in school language study, perhaps because its obliqueness is often sophisticated and in consequence eludes the understanding of many learners until they are well into teenage years. Wilkie Collins's *The Moonstone* used to be set for public English examinations. The First Narrative in the Second Period of that detective story is contributed by the outrageous Drusilla Clack. Her eighty pages are based on the diary she had meticulously kept. Adult readers hardly need the warning (through the mouth of the house-steward, Gabriel Betteredge) that she is a very unreliable witness. The author, with heavy irony, makes her talk with revolting unctuousness. She prates ('clacks'!) relentlessly about her 14 clerical friends, about her distribution of moral tracts reprinted from the chapters of a 'famous' work entitled *The Serpent at Home*. These tracts have titles like 'Satan in the Hair Brush', 'Satan under the Table', and so on. She also refers repeatedly to her charitable work for the Mothers' Small Clothes Conversion Society which rescued unredeemed fathers' trousers from pawnbrokers and 'abridged' them for issue to mothers with small sons. Her blatant self-satisfaction has been missed (despite her surname) by some 16-year-old candidates, otherwise quite intelligent, who, when invited to write about Miss Clack, took her and her remorseless 'Christian' virtues literally and at face value. It could hardly have been only examination conditions that accounted for their unawareness of the ironical undercurrent.

Principles and maxims

It is not necessary for teachers to adopt and use any formal categorization of the pragmatic features of language such as academic linguists are currently engaged on. Teachers do not need in their job to master the somewhat forbidding terminology of themes and rhemes, of right-branching, of logical implicatures and entailments, and so on. Nevertheless, the territory that this terminology maps, focusing predominantly on ordinary conversation and personal communicative exchanges and discussions, and therefore very much on spoken language, has come increasingly to be recognized as central to subject-English as well as to language across the curriculum. The British educational system notoriously concedes teaching importance only to subjects or areas that achieve public examination status. Despite doubts about the dominant roles of examining, testing and assessment within the whole educational process, one must welcome the rating of English as one of the National Curriculum's three foundation core subjects and the firm placing of spoken English (oral skills) in the forefront of sets of standard attainment tasks (SATs). If competence in spoken English is (belatedly) to be taken more seriously and to be given more classroom attention than hitherto, teachers – not just of English – will need to become more aware of pragmatic factors that influence the 'balance of power' between speakers and hearers as well as between writers and readers.

In tackling language use from the linguist's point of view, Leech's Interpersonal Rhetoric establishes a Cooperative Principle (CP) and a Politeness Principle (PP). His CP distinguishes four of the maxims listed in his diagram (Figure 7). Adapted from Grice (1957, 377–88), these are four precepts for successful communication:

Quantity: Give the right amount of information.
Quality: Try to make your contribution one that is true.
Relation: Be relevant.
Manner: Be perspicuous (specifically avoid obscurity of expression; avoid ambiguity; be brief; be orderly).

Leech (1983, Chapter 4) gives many examples of utterances, both 'monologue' sentences and exchanges. He explains and interprets the meaning of each – both the surface meaning and the 'semantic susurrus'. A few of his examples, plus one or two others, may be quoted to illustrate his method. Thus:

A: We'll all miss Bill and Agatha, won't we?
B: Well, we'll all miss Bill.

Here B fails to satisfy the Maxim of Quantity by confirming only one part of A's opinion. By implication (technically 'implicature') B suggests that 'we'll not miss Agatha'. Had he explicitly said so, he would have breached the PP by being impolite.

The Irony Principle operates in

A: Geoff has just borrowed your car.
B: Well, I like *that*!

Obviously B is not being literally truthful (he did *not* like it) but retains the semblance of being polite to Geoff. Other implicatures are demonstrated with

'Employees do not have to retire at 65', implying that 'Employees *can* retire at 65'. Similarly, 'Frank tried to open the door' implies that he did not succeed.

Entailment is obvious in 'Sally is *the* secretary', because necessarily 'Sally is *a* secretary'. In this construction the definite article 'the' actually expresses a degree of definiteness. This contrasts with 'I won a prize today', which implies that the receiver of the message does not know *which* prize (was it first, second or third?) is being referred to – it is left indefinite. Another related example, quoted from Clark and Clark (1977, p. 122) shows mischievously how what is logically true can pragmatically be very misleading:

Steven: Wilfrid is meeting a woman for dinner tonight.
Susan: Does his wife know about it?
Steven: Of course she does. The woman he is meeting is his wife.

Sometimes an illocution conceals beneath a subsidiary surface question a more significant *intended* question:

A: Can you tell me the time?
B: Yes.

The concealed question, deliberately overlooked by a perverse interlocutor intent upon scoring a pseudo-logical point, is then revealed:

A: Well, what is it?

A last example can easily be shown in a sentence such as: '*Wuthering Heights* was not written by Jane Austen.' Compared with the positively worded '*Wuthering Heights* was written by Emily Brontë', the former is, in Leech's phrase, an example of 'negative uninformativeness'. Not that all negative statements are unhelpful in this way. Where only two alternatives – one positive, one negative – are feasible, both are equally informative, as in 'My pet dog is not female / is male', but such clear-cut polarized pairs are less common than multiple possibilities; 'not all', for example, may oppose either 'all' or 'some' by meaning 'a few' or a different 'some'.

The increasing emphasis on 'communicative competence', especially in the teaching of foreign languages, promises a more balanced treatment of semantics, discourse and other pragmatics of language. If, in response to the Kingman Report (DES, 1988), some kind of reinstatement of language study is achieved in the teaching of English as a first language and if a 'return to grammar' is not a return to traditional quasi-Latin grammar, there is reason to hope that any new pedagogical grammar will pay realistic attention to semantics and pragmatics. There are, of course, many other features of 'pragmalinguistics' than those discussed in this chapter, but a few of them will be touched upon in a consideration of discourse theory in the next chapter.

9

The two-layered code – discourse

All discourses but my own afflict me; they seem hard, impertinent and irksome.

(Ben Jonson)

Conversation

In a book suggestively titled *Language, Sense and Nonsense*, two philosophers reported Frege's view of language as 'rife with vagueness'. They themselves choose the utterance 'How does language work?' as an example of 'some hopelessly vague question' (Baker and Hacker, 1984, p. 372). A few years later, the Kingman Committee was required to confront that 'vague' question in relation to the teaching of the English language. The Committee's terms of reference implied that 'how the English language works' could be adequately described and that 'what, in general terms, pupils had to know about how the English language works' could be specified. Their report (DES, 1988) produced (as we noted earlier, p. 12) a 'model' which segments our language into parts:

1 Forms
2 (i) Communication
   (ii) Comprehension
3 Acquisition and development
4 Historical and geographical variation.

Practical considerations – determined by governmental policy or tactics – made simplification such as this understandable, perhaps inevitable. Nevertheless, to separate the many dimensions, while suiting the convenience of describing language, is less suited to the teaching and learning of language. It contributes to what has been attacked (with some justice as well as some exaggeration) as the 'striking dimensionality shrinkage of modern linguistics'. The professor of general linguistics who made this observation goes on to amplify his accusation: 'Once linguistic theory, by decontextualising language, insists on reduction to a simple plane of "form", a single plane of "meaning", and a single scale of "grammaticality", whole landscapes of linguistic nuance have already been flattened out by descriptive bulldozing' (Harris, 1987, p. 152).

Communication is only one of the uses of language but it is a large and very complex one, especially in the sphere of education. There, it focuses, or should focus, particularly on interpersonal functions. For teachers, language lessons – in so far as they can be distinguished from the more purely personal concerns of literature – need to concentrate, as Sinclair (1985) says, less on 'a single stream of speech or writing' and more on 'a two-layered code' of conversations that involve 'constantly checking, evaluating, summarising, labelling, scene-setting, etc.'.

Whether linguistics has become, as it were, less severely linguistic by expanding to include language behaviour once thought to lie outside its boundaries is a matter of terminological labelling. Those dedicated to a strict linguistics that is highly specialized, scientific and rigorous may deny the title to anything but their own 'pure' discipline. They may leave other areas that have developed later and seem to have become 'growth areas' to be called applied or pedagogical or historical linguistics, or child language acquisition – or discourse analysis. Coulthard, who – with Sinclair – took the lead in the innovatory study of discourse analysis, begins his *Introduction* with a testimony that Firth, a pioneer English linguist, regarded conversation as a central topic in linguistics, though for years not taken to be such: 'it is now forty years since J. R. Firth urged linguists to study conversation, for "it is here that we shall find the key to a better understanding of what language is and how it works"' (Coulthard, 1977, p. 1).

The expansion of the study of language has tended to make the term 'linguistic' unduly elastic. (The suggestion that a new adjective, 'lingual' – the basic morpheme of 'bilingual' and 'multilingual' – could distinguish *language*-relatedness from *linguistics*-relatedness, has not been widely adopted.) In consequence, some teachers of English have allowed their antipathy to narrowly defined linguistics to reject broader interpretations that involve *all* language behaviour – including conversation, even desultory conversation or 'chat'. Even Iris Murdoch's Julius (in *A Fairly Honourable Defeat*), who defined language as 'a reasonably useful jumble with an in-built capacity to manoeuvre itself', might (via his creator) have conceded that his remark belonged only marginally to linguistics in the extended sense. In fact, the pragmatics dimension has blurred the borderline between the linguistic and the non-linguistic by accepting 'perlocutions'. Coulthard (1977, p. 18) makes this point clearly in arguing that while 'Basically an illocutionary act is a linguistic act performed in uttering certain words in a given context, a perlocutionary act is a *non-linguistic* act performed as a consequence of the locutionary and illocutionary acts.'

Traditionally, and to some extent still (as we noted from the beginning, p. 3), teaching about English language has largely meant teaching grammar and/or teaching literature. Both restrictions on total 'English' have been found unsatisfactory. They have both concentrated too much on the written, the approved language variety and the literary, and too little on the spoken, the less prestigious varieties and the non-literary. This imbalance is gradually being redressed, largely by acceptance of all kinds of discourse as worthy of attention and as bridging the gulf between school language, 'schoolmastered' language, street language and home language, between formal grammar and functional-semantic grammar, between isolated, uncontextualized language and 'situationed' language, between linguistic order, commonly confined to single short sentences, and the untidy disorder of much supra-sentential language. If, as Lady Welby (1903, p. 78), with typical forcefulness, observed nearly a century ago, 'we think in specks and lumps of stuff; we must learn to think in throb and complex whirl or intricate convolution', then we must learn to converse in similarly varied ways.

James Moffett has written a valuable book on *Teaching the Universe of Discourse* (1968). He arranges kinds of discourse in order of 'increasing distance between speaker and audience, between first and second person'. By stretching 'discourse' to cover thinking or talking to oneself, he includes in his four categories the *intra*personal as well as the *inter*personal and the *im*personal (Moffett, 1968, p. 33):

1 Reflection – intrapersonal communication between two parts of one nervous system.
2 Conversation – interpersonal communication between two people in vocal range.
3 Correspondence – interpersonal communication between remote individuals or small groups with some personal knowledge of each other.
4 Publication – impersonal communication to a larger anonymous group extended over space and/or time.

With 'a little tautological transforming' of himself, he relates this sequence to a parallel four 'traditional categories of discourse – drama, narrative, exposition and argumentation'. Redefining these 'in terms of (1) distance between speaker and subject, (2) levels of abstraction, and (3) a sequence of activities or skills which the student should learn how to do', he lists:

what is happening – drama – recording
what happened   – narrative – reporting
what happens   – exposition – generalizing
what may happen – logical argumentation – theorizing
(ibid., pp. 35–6)

Conversational discourse – Moffett's number (2) in the list (above) – is restricted to spoken exchanges between two people. In ordinary language it extends to similar exchanges among small groups of people but, when more speakers are involved, it breaks up into fragments of discourse, that is, conversations. The dramatis personae in a play are not in the usual sense conversing, though a small number may simulate spontaneous conversation. That the few actors engaged may (and usually do) repeat the words of a written text makes their quasi-conversation correspond in present time (what is happening) to fictional reports of a past time (what has happened). The language used in such conversing as occurs in plays and in prose fiction (Ivy Compton-Burnett's novels rely almost entirely on conversation) is more or less remote from ordinary colloquial language. It has often been pointed out that it would be intolerable to hear actors speak or to read aloud the utterances of fictional characters as if their words corresponded exactly to the language of actual everyday conversation. All kinds of discourse, including exposition, generalizing and logical argumentation as well as drama, journals, biographies, essays, etc., can of course be, as it were, topics of meta-communication. A language-awareness course should recognize the gaps and differences separating the various forms of discourse as well as the features that link them. The basic uses of language are, as Suzanne Langer says (1962, p. 33), 'question and answer, assertion and denial, denotation and description'. All these modes – and others – operate in all the exchanges mentioned.

Classroom discourse

In principle, academic discourse analysis could chart conversational interplay of various types in various contexts. The conversations analysed could have taken place, for example, in doctors' surgeries, alongside psychiatrists' couches, at interviews for appointments, in homes (where mothers and children often converse), in headmasters' studies – and, of course, in school classrooms. In fact, most systematic analysis has been made of doctor–patient consultations, of mother–infant conversation, and of school classroom discourse. For educational purposes we are less concerned with medical exchanges, more with pre-school parent–child talk, and most of all with classroom interaction. In comparatively recent years, a large and growing academic 'industry' has developed for investigating child language acquisition, especially in the pre-school period. The existence of learned periodicals such as the *Journal of Child Language* testifies to the size, complexity and importance of the work. It must suffice here to mention one very relevant finding established by Gordon Wells (1974) and referred to by Britton (1977, p. 15):

> In the material so far analyzed, Wells has found that 70 per cent of the verbal interactions are initiated not by the mother but by the child. School, on this score, must seem a whole new ball game to the first grader!

This sharp contrast, in percentage terms probably unexpected, derives, no doubt, from the different contextual situations. The very young child acquires a large amount of his/her language competence from the opportunities of balanced reciprocal interchanges with a parent, more usually with a mother. Comparably 'natural' opportunities may to some degree extend into nursery and pre-school situations and even sometimes – in fortunate circumstances – into the first years of compulsory education, but are likely to diminish quickly and progressively as 'unnatural' school conditions tend to prevail, with larger classes taught more and more as homogeneous units. Small-group work may be more common today than it was fifty years ago, but it seems not to have become a dominant teaching method. An anthology of the 92 observational classroom systems described by

Simon and Boyer (1967) presents analyses predominantly of interactions between single teachers and whole classes. After a decade or so of studying many of
the remarkably numerous systems being tried out, one critic (a scholar in the
University of Liège) judged the results to be still unimpressive, though he looked
forward to more promising results:

> However weak the present classroom interaction analysis systems may still be, one is
> more and more convinced that they will play a tremendous role in the improvement
> of actual school practice by revealing it as it really is, and not as teachers or
> educationists think or dream it is.
>
>   (G. de Landsheere, in Chanan (ed.), 1973, p. 81)

Given the many variables affecting school practice, generalization can only be
impressionistic. Schools differ considerably in a multitude of ways; they differ in
their language-teaching arrangements, in relationships between teachers of
native and teachers of foreign languages, in attitudes to language across the
curriculum, in teachers' personal uses of language and judgements about their
students' language use, and indeed about their own language behaviour. One
reputable non-educationist writer has ventured the opinion that the only safe
generalization to make about teaching is that all teachers talk too much. Analysis
of classroom discourse seems to support that criticism. According to the
oft-quoted Flanders Two-Thirds Rule, based on data supplied by 147 teachers
from all grade levels (presumably in the USA):

> About two-thirds of the time spent in a classroom, someone is talking. The chances
> are about two out of three that this person is the teacher. When the teacher talks,
> two-thirds of the time is spent in many expressions of opinion and fact, giving some
> directions, and occasionally criticising the pupils'. (Flanders, in Amidon and Hough,
> 1987, p. 285)

Drawing on an earlier Flanders document (1963), Wragg says (in Chanan, 1973,
p. 92) that 'For teachers rated "poor" he [Flanders] had found a rule of
three-quarters was more the norm'. Flanders's results also showed apparently
that 'student achievement is higher in the classes of teachers who used more
indirect influence and that teachers who use more direct influence do not vary
their behaviour in different situations as much as the "indirect" teachers'
(Davies, 1977, pp. 171–2).

The observers doing research into classroom discourse used various systems
categorizing the verbal actions involved. The Flanders (1970, p. 34) method,
using Flanders's Interaction Analysis Categories, divided up each lesson into
three-second units, assigning them to ten headed sections. Teacher Talk was
distributed among

1 accepting feelings
2 praising or encouraging
3 accepting or using pupils' ideas
4 asking questions

5 lecturing
6 giving directions
7 criticizing or justifying authority

(1–3 being classified as response events, 5–7 as initiations events) and Pupil Talk was subdivided into

8 response
9 initiation
10 silence or confusion.

The numbering implied no scale, it merely designated the classes.

Bellack *et al.* (1966), using transcripts, classified the verbal actions of students and teachers into four major categories. What they called 'pedagogical moves' were labelled as structuring, soliciting, responding, reacting. They found, not surprisingly, that teachers were considerably more verbally active than their pupils. Teachers controlled three of the four pedagogical moves. By dominating the one remaining move – responding – they left each pupil 'a very limited role to play in classroom discussions'. Researchers concluded that 'the core of classroom discourse is the response-expectant soliciting move followed by the expectancy-fulfilling move'.

In England, classroom language was investigated during the 1970s at the University of Birmingham by a team led by Sinclair and Coulthard (who had earlier examined doctor–patient language). Their report (Sinclair *et al.*, 1972) presented a model of classroom analysis that divided discourse into *exchanges* which comprised *moves* and *acts* building up into *transactions* and *lessons*. A typical classroom exchange structure, they reported (in somewhat awkward phrasing), 'consists of an *Initiation* by the teacher, followed by a *Response* from the pupil, followed by *Feedback*, to the pupil's [*sic*] response from the teacher' (Sinclair *et al.*, 1972, pp. 64–5, 72). This sequence came to be abbreviated to IRF and is illustrated in Coulthard's (1977, p. 106) subsequent *Introduction to Discourse Analysis* (mentioned above, p. 100) by a chart of an actual 'eliciting exchange':

initiating move	Can anyone have a shot, guess at that one?	(elicit)
responding move	Cleopatra	(reply)
follow-up move	Cleopatra	(accept)
	Good girl She was the most famous queen, wasn't she?	(evaluation) (comment)

A very thorough and up-to-date survey of systems of classroom observation has been presented by Edwards and Westgate (1987). They emphasize the limitations of all forms of recording, which are unavoidably selective and partial.

While recognizing *spoken* language as 'the vital medium for communication and learning', they also accept uncertainty in interpreting surface talk arising from 'a fundamental variability in the relationship between linguistic forms and their functions in discourse'. In particular, they emphasize 'the high degree of obliqueness and indeterminacy which characterizes conversation, and which also marks a good deal of talk even in more formal, institutionalized settings like classrooms' (Edwards and Westgate, 1987, p. 178).

Classroom discourse analysis provides descriptions of what, in terms of language, actually often happens in lessons. The objective descriptions of patterns of language behaviour do not coincide exactly with what teachers think happens (or with what ought to happen). Experimental evidence has proved that many teachers seriously underestimate how much they talk. In so far as much of their talk is 'directive', they tend to dominate. Messer calls the classroom language controlled by teachers, 'a sort of shadow language'. The study which he reports has

> confirmed my own experience that, rather than being good, effective, or of a higher standard than the children's own language, [teacher-controlled classroom language] is in fact a sort of shadow language often echoing little of their real language potential. This 'good' level which many teachers strive to cultivate in children is in fact of an impoverished and depressed standard compared to what is actually available. (In Torbe & Protherough (eds) 1976, p. 89)

Another severe critic, writing in the context of second-language teaching, points out:

> The language of the classroom and the language of each subject tend to be a special register, distinct from the expressive talk which the child normally employs. By rejecting such expressive talk, and by using new and unfamiliar registers, the teacher defines the rules by which the classroom game is to be played. (White, 1974, p. 129)

The transcriptions of lessons by Barnes *et al.* (1969) illustrate the games 'played' in biology, religious education, science, chemistry, physics, history, mathematics and geography. In these lessons teachers can impose their preconceived structures; sometimes they insist on what Creber famously called 'playing teacher's word game' – for example, when requiring a 'pseudo-question' (presumably in a religious education lesson about Rebecca at the well) to be answered with the exact word 'pitcher'. The discourse mapped by researchers into classroom language contains little that can be readily described as conversation, as expressive talk or as 'two-layered' in the normal understanding of these terms. Stubbs (1976, p. 99) accepts the question-answer-evaluation sequence as a 'common conversational structure' but even so equates it with a 'riddle' where 'the pupils have to guess what particular word or expression the teacher is thinking of'. Had the Flanders analysis (pp. 103–4 above) refined his item 4 – teacher's questioning – by at least separating 'closed' from 'open' questions, he would presumably also have found a shortage of open questions.

Barnes (1971, pp. 74–5), who had valuably used the open/closed distinction, expanded his earlier statements about 'Teachers' Awareness of Language' (p. 22 above) by more specifically arguing that teachers need

(a) to develop a more sophisticated insight into the implications of the language they themselves use, especially the 'language of secondary education';
(b) to study the possibilities that the 'gulf' between teacher and pupil hinders learning because of the specialist terminology used;
(c) to look more closely at the role of language in learning new concepts;
(d) to study closed and open questions and the value of discussion;
(e) to become more aware of implicit teaching objectives;
(f) to make explicit to pupils the criteria by which their performance will be accepted or rejected.

These recommendations are directed, of course, at teachers of all subjects. But of particular relevance to teachers of languages, native and foreign, are the emphases (in (d) and (f)) on the value of discussion and on making explicit the criteria applied in judging performances. Question–answer sequences, as near to discussion or conversation as many lessons achieve, raise queries about relationships between grammatical and communicative criteria, which often diverge. Moffett (1968, p. 78) is persuasive in submitting that 'the most important and successful way we learn linguistic forms is by internalizing the whole give and take of conversation'. It is perhaps easier to accommodate this recommendation in first-language teaching, where 'give' and 'take' are more readily balanced, than in foreign-language teaching, where responses may be grammatically correct but communicatively unnatural or odd.

We cannot but accept that 'It is difficult to imagine how a naturally communicative use of speech could possibly be reproduced in classroom conditions' (Davies and Widdowson, 1974, p. 162). Nevertheless, it is desirable for teachers of languages – first, second or foreign – to make conditions as favourable as possible for 'natural' expressive language use in real or quasi-real simulated conversation. In spite of the triumph of 'communicative competence' over drill exercises – especially (though by no means exclusively) in methods of teaching foreign languages – too much time can still be spent on speaking in grammatically full sentences and practising structures that are technically 'correct' but semantically and behaviourally unlikely. Only the pseudo-conversation of the classroom generates exchanges translated into an English lacking normal pronominalizations and ellipsis, as in:

'What is that under your arm?'
'It is a tennis racquet.'
'Where did you find that racquet?'
'I found this racquet in the cupboard under the stairs.'

Ordinary spoken English would use more abbreviations ('*It's* a . . .'), more pronouns ('. . . find *it*'), and more ellipsis ([I found it] 'In the cupboard under the stairs') but at least the exchange is about a real event. By contrast, as Coulthard (1977, p. 139) reports,

> it has been suggested, only semi-humorously, that one result of introducing foreign students to the present continuous in English with appropriate actions, 'I am opening the window', 'I am cleaning the board', is to create the impression that one of the quirks of English is to keep commenting on what they are doing.

Communicative competence

It is not possible to consider in any detail the impact of 'communicative' pedagogical techniques on the teaching of foreign languages, but there seems to have been a marked movement towards greater emphasis on speaking, on using ordinary language in more nearly authentic situations, and on more balanced exchanges in small groups and student pairs. This movement has been strengthened by increased use of role-play and simulations. All these developments must have stimulated more fluent conversational discourse. A series of research projects funded by the Scottish Education Department has produced *Communicative Language Teaching in Practice* (Mitchell, 1988). The author found that 'a large majority [of teachers of foreign languages] claimed to be doing some form of non-whole-class work reasonably regularly' and that 'It seemed taken for granted that such sessions be given over to oral work' (Mitchell, 1988, p. 39).

The gulf between foreign- and native-language teaching – in Britain between FLT and EL1T (teaching English as a first language) – has been narrowing conspicuously. Developments in linguistic and pedagogical theory and the growing presence in schools of pupils needing to acquire English as a second or foreign language (E2L, EFL) have reduced the insularity of English as a native language (ENL) and placed it more firmly in a multilingual and multicultural context. These considerations will surely complicate problems caused by the testing of spoken English being made a compulsory component for GCSE. Without entering the vexed arguments about whether spoken English can be satisfactorily evaluated at all and, if it can, whether such evaluation is feasible at the age of 16, past experience of oral English assessments implies that conversation will be a significant feature and that much conversation will be of the small-group kind. In preparation specifically for this, teachers will surely need to be aware – and to make their students aware – of the characteristics and complexities of good conversation.

Teachers in multicultural societies need, or at least may benefit from, work done on the ethnography of speaking, much of which has concentrated on formal dimensions and has described in structural terms language behaviour that is well defined, sometimes ritualized, in various communities, for example, modes of greeting, ritual insults and 'rapping' games. Less specialized and of more general interest to all teachers are features revealed and charted by the analysis of more ordinary conversation. One basic feature of such conversation is that of 'turn-taking'. Though pupils normally appreciate in theory that in conversation each interlocutor adopts alternatively the role of speaker and that of listener, in practice they often break the conventional rules by talking simultaneously. Even sixth-formers aiming at university entrance need to be warned – especially in test conditions – against excessive 'overlapping' by speakers, against 'queuing up' to speak in turn, against an individual monopolizing too much of the time available, against failing to draw into the discussion a reluctant member of the group, against undue silence between 'turns'. They need to become overtly aware of the appropriate register and of the value of maintaining relevance and progression. They might benefit from becoming conscious of the paralinguistic and kinesic cues that, along with intonational and grammatical indications, give signals that control the conversational process.

For social purposes – outside the school and the assessment situation – many of these factors (though, of course, not body-language behaviour) might usefully be studied in relation to telephone conversation. Questions of who speaks first when the receiver's phone is lifted and of how identities and modes of address are established can be contrasted with the routines and conventions observed in foreign countries.

The sum total of language interaction, involving a complex network of linguistic, social and interpersonal dimensions, constitutes a large part of language awareness.

10 Translation

> The earliest and still one of the best roads to linguistic
> understanding is through the comparison of one language with
> another.
>
> (Dwight Bolinger)

A persistent problem in discussing language awareness is that so much depends on what exactly is meant by 'language'. This word can be parsed as a count-noun, which (in English) is either singular in number (*a* language), or plural (language*s*), or as an abstract mass-noun, which – without a determiner – is normally singular (*L*anguage). Approaches to language awareness sometimes work 'from the bottom upwards', starting with particular languages and moving towards universal qualities shared by all languages. Approaches of this kind risk the 'creative untidiness' already mentioned (Preface and p. 13). Had the strong version of the Whorf–Sapir hypothesis (cf. p. 32) been validated and each language could be shown to *determine* meanings, there would presumably be no 'top' of language universals to be reached 'from the bottom up'. Approaches from the opposite direction, 'from the top down', would start from theoretical universals and seek to substantiate them in particular languages. This seems tidier and more logical, but encounters controversies about whether and to what extent there really are universal features shared by the many thousands of languages that exist.

The member of HMI who dismissed full language-awareness courses as 'panaceas currently in vogue' conceded cautiously, even tentatively, that 'there may be a case for taster courses'. But these 'should leave the main [foreign] language courses intact'. The planning associated with language-awareness courses should, in his view, 'involve the co-operation of at least the English and modern languages departments' (p. 24). Whether such modest changes (already achieved in some schools) can reasonably be expected to raise standards of competence in using languages (foreign or native) is very questionable. Standards in foreign languages attained by native English speakers compare unfavourably with those achieved by foreigners, especially European foreigners, learning English or indeed other languages.

The complex nature of languages makes it difficult to find 'hard' evidence that awareness of more than one language is educationally essential or even desirable. Nevertheless, the experience and judgements presented in a formidable number of reports, papers and books published since the middle of the nineteenth century cannot be dismissed as mere 'vested interest' matters. The arguments collated by James (1979) draw on publications listed in a table of references filling more than two pages. From the Taunton Report of 1868 he quotes the firm assertion that 'There can be no doubt that a boy [*sic*!] gains very much in the study of his own language by the study of another'. Much more recently, the Association of Teachers of Russian in 1977 submitted (to the NCLE's working party on Foreign Languages in Education) a claim for 'the place of modern languages in general and of Russian in the curriculum of educational establishments in Britain.' From this, James noted that 'a number of writers see the unique contribution provided by language learning at school as an awakening within the pupil of a conceptual awareness of language'. He linked it with the view, expressed in 1972 by the Scottish Central Committee for Modern Languages, that language learning provided 'a general linguistic training which will give the pupil a surer appreciation of the value of words and help him to use his own language more effectively by showing him how language in general works' (James, 1979, p. 10).

Textual substitution

It is in this connection that translation becomes relevant. The problems it raises – and they are considerable – often turn on the question of whether linguistic form and linguistic meaning are wrongly (though conveniently) treated as separable. If they could be separated, then translation could be regarded as a mechanical process replacing one set of textual counters in the original language by an equivalent set from a target language. This formal operation allowed Colin Cherry (1957, p. 177) to maintain that 'machine translation is of course not concerned with "meaning" at all in our present sense of that word, not with meaning *to* someone, but purely with "syntactic transformation" – textual substitutions from an original to a target language'. When Harris (1987, p. 80) describes processes of textual substitution as 'blind', he perhaps had in mind the oft-quoted account of the computer translation of 'out of sight, out of mind' into 'blind idiot'. Though this story is often now regarded as amusing but apocryphal, it was reported earlier, and with circumstantial detail, as actually happening at an international conference in Delhi. A woman MP from Rochester, it was said, used the same proverb in her speech. It 'duly disappeared into the maw of umpteen Asiatic translators' and she 'got a translation of a translation back later, rendering it as "invisible idiot"'. Perhaps the machines produced two rather different transformations of 'out of sight'. The two programs reveal the unexpected formal ambiguity that conceals the semantic distinction between the idiomatic 'beyond (my) mind's eye' and the literal 'lacking (eye)sight'.

A similar computer translation allegedly (and less plausibly) turned 'The spirit is willing but the flesh is weak' into the target-language equivalent of 'The vodka is good but the meat is lousy'. Computers do more effectively (and more speedily) what human mistranslators have often performed with traditional pen-and-paper equipment. Among the countless examples of mistranslated ambiguity that are on record, it is naturally the amusing and 'suggestive' ones that are most easily remembered and most often quoted. A favourite short item has been the Portuguese advertisement of a 'SHADY HOTEL'. Franglais has a Far Eastern rival in the 'Japlish' language, conflating Japanese and English. A Japanese with some knowledge of English is said to have translated the Japanese constitution's equivalent of 'Life, liberty and the pursuit of happiness' into 'Licence to commit lustful pleasure'. The wishful thinking by which one wants this to be credible might also add plausibility to the report that a cablegram sent to Russia announcing 'Genevieve suspended for prank' was rendered into Russian and then back into English as 'Genevieve hanged for juvenile delinquency'.

One of our most inventively humorous writers – Paul Jennings – exploits translation as a source of amusement. But, amid the delightfully rich data he uses, hints of serious concerns come briefly to the surface and provoke reflection on issues which it is not his business to pursue. A short piece on 'Beatrix Potter Translated' (anthologized in Potter, 1954) begins: 'It is difficult to decide whether translators are heroes or fools.' Is the translator a superior being who

> floats over the world in a god-like balloon? The battle of voices under the arches of teeming cities, the infinite variations of uvula and hard palate, the words formed in tribal battles and in tales over the winter hearth, float up to him in a vague, jumbled unity, rich but disembodied, like a distant cooking smell.

Have 'the racial realities of language' become for him 'mere intellectual concepts'? It is surely unfortunate that 'the children in the village, who have one language and one vision', will not see the European characters named by translators of Beatrix Potter. At most, they will catch a glimpse, from behind the dimity curtains of their homes in the Potter village, of an international procession. Among the personalities passing and momentarily caught sight of will be 'the awful Mauriac Famille Flopsaut' (Flopsy Bunnies), the gaudy Noisy-Noisette, the Mata Hari of the twenties (Squirrel Nutkin) and the Maupassant Pêche-à-la-Ligne (Jeremy Fisher), a 'quiet angler who pushes his mistress's husband into the trout pool'. From Germany comes die Hasenfamilie Plumps (more Flopsy Bunnies) and Frau Tigge-Winkel (Mrs Tiggy-Winkle). Italy is represented by Il Coniglio Pierino (Peter Rabbit), imagined by Jennings as 'a swarthy Sicilian bandit'. Curiously, though, from geographically nearer Wales, Jemima Puddle-Duck is linguistically the least recognizable as Hanes Dili Minnlyn.

It is, as Jennings comments, a paradox that 'the more a work expresses some special national genius, the more it attracts translators'. Until he discovered the translations of Beatrix Potter, he had regarded 'Jabberwocky' as the supreme example of an Englishness in language that captivates foreigners. He greatly admires the French and German versions, reprinted in Gardner's *The Annotated Alice* (1970), and quotes from one of the Latin versions ('even Latin') the line 'ensis vorpalis persnicuit persnacuitque' ('The vorpal blade went snicker-snack').

It is doubtful whether machine translation has yet managed to cope with

'Jabberwocky'. Harris quotes, from a book about machine translation, an example which illustrates the shortcomings of non-semantic 'textual substitution'. Presumably for technical reasons, the French marks of accent are printed as numerical digits in the following:

AVANT-PROPOS

PRE1SENTER AU LECTEUR QUI N EST SPE1CIALISE1 NI DANS L E1TUDE DE LA LINGUISTIQUE NI DANS LA CONNAISSANCE DES CALCULATRICES E1LECTRONIQUES, LES PROBLE2MES ACTUELS DE LA TRADUCTION AUTOMATIQUE DES LANGUES, TEL EST LE BUT DANS LEQUEL CE LIVRE A E1TE1 CONCU.

In English, this becomes:

BEFORE-REMARK

TO PRESENT AT THE READER WHICH IS SPECIALISED NEITHER IN THE STUDY OF THE LINGUISTIC NOR IN THE KNOWLEDGE OF THE AUTOMATIC TRADUCTION OF THE LANGUAGES, SUCH IS THE AIM IN WHICH THIS BOOK HAD BEEN CONCEIVED.

Harris (1987, pp. 83–4) comments that 'the English version reads remarkably like the effort of a French beginner struggling to master English in the early stages of learning that language'. It would be rash, however, to think on this evidence that computers are not already doing better and will not one day cope even with the most idiomatic wordings.

Caution and reported experience warn us not to underrate the enormous complexities of all non-literal language, even within a single language. A Yale University machine was set, not to translate English into a second language, but merely to condense reports in English about earthquakes. So completely did its shortening overlook the details supplied that it produced 'There was an earthquake in America today' from a story which began with 'The death of the Pope shook America today' (Campbell, 1982). Our current technology is as yet (and perhaps may long remain) unable satisfactorily to change versions – either by shortening or by translating – without acquiring the capacity to think. In the words of Umberto Eco (1976, Preface), a semiologist as well as a novelist of considerable repute, 'To re-write in another language means to *re-think*'. Machines, as yet unable to think, can only transliterate, though admittedly that can be a useful service.

In 1988 the quinquennial World Congress of Philosophy speculated at a high theoretical level on its theme of 'The Philosophical Understanding of Human Beings'. Lord Elton, as chairman, recalled that the philosopher Schleiermacher had said that every language was a particular mode of thought and could not be repeated in the same way in any other language. Since Schleiermacher almost certainly had written in German, it follows that, if his (Schleiermacher's) statement is true, it was not made by Schleiermacher. Conversely, if it was made by him, then this is not what he said!

A more practical problem affected a distinguished English professor of French. Invited to address a learned audience in Paris, he is supposed to have taken the precaution of sending his script to a French colleague. The Englishman wanted to be sure that his use of what was still for him a second language was linguistically impeccable. The Frenchman replied with a list of 'corrections' of phrases which were not quite 'natural' French and should be replaced by slightly different usages. The English professor conceded that the revisions might be more 'French' than the originals, but rejected them because they did not say exactly what he meant. He was in effect confirming the neat Italian proverb 'Traduttore, traditore' ('A translator is a traitor'). The inevitability of this 'treachery' derives from the fact that different languages, even closely related European languages, are not completely isomorphic. At various levels, they lack exact one-to-one correspondences. In a recent article entitled 'Who Will Translate the Translators', Harris (1989) contrasts a hypothetical situation – 'If all languages were structurally isomorphic, there would simply be no translation dilemma' – with the reality in which

> languages A, B, C, D, E . . . are related in such a way that, to evoke a photographic metaphor, each seems to be a slightly blurred version of the other . . . The Euroglot community has for centuries been a community of that order, sharing a set of languages all cut to roughly the same cognitive pattern (which Benjamin Lee Whorf later christened 'Standard Average European') . . .

The qualifying phrases – 'slightly blurred', 'roughly the same' – pinpoint the approximate character of all translation between different languages and even, probably, between different dialects of recognizably the same language. At best – quoting the clever winning entry in a competition to explain 'How do Translators Do It?' – 'Translators Do It With Cunning, Lingually', that is, with maximum equivalence.

Cultural variation

A reviewer of a conference on machine translation has commented that 'Translators . . . live in an uncomfortable no-man's land between two languages, where the differences between cultures loom large' (Salkie, 1989, p. vi). Obviously, because linguistic differences are embedded in cultural differences, degrees and kinds of difficulty in translation vary considerably. Where a difference is simply physical or concrete, a loan-word (such as 'sari' or 'muezzin') is transferred without translation. The same is reasonably possible with more abstract terms referring to behaviour (such as 'leitmotiv' in discussing music or 'langlauf' in talking about ski-ing). A curious exchange allows English to use 'palais de dance' when French prefers 'le dancing'. But some words seem untranslatable and the borrowed equivalent depends on clarification of the concept from context, as with 'droit de seigneur' or with 'touché' (when used metaphorically in argument). Emotions can defy satisfactory translation between languages; German 'Gemüt-lichkeit', enjoyed particularly 'après ski', is only partially captured by 'sociability' or 'joviality', while French 'joie de vivre' is more vivacious than the stodgier 'joy of living'. It was the unhappy association of English 'wild' with French 'sauvage' that caused the World Wildlife Fund to be renamed the World-wide Fund for Nature. The answer to the teasing question posed by Bolinger (1975, p. 266) – 'Does the fact that South Americans call a screwdriver a *tornillador* ('screw-driver') while Spaniards call it a *destornillador* ('screw-remover') prove that South Americans are more constructive?' – is presumably 'no'. A trivial linguistic detail cannot be expected to *prove* anything about the users. But the fact that the question can even be asked raises much bigger problems about the complex relationships between language and culture. In a multicultural society such as Britain's, language awareness depends on cultural awareness. The National Curriculum consultation document (DES and Welsh Office, 1987) and the consequent official documents on implementing its requirements for English have, not surprisingly, elicited criticisms of its restrictedly insular Anglicity (cf. Brumfit, 1988, p. 9). The President of the Confederation of Indian Organiz-ations (UK) – Tara Mukherjee – welcomes 'the prominence given to foreign languages in the secondary curriculum' but is none the less organizing a national campaign against 'the inadvertent marginalisation of Indic languages'. It is difficult to deny the insistence that

> All children need to develop a firm linguistic base in their first language before attempting to learn a second language. Confidence is a prerequisite for all learning, but the Government's rejection of the child's total linguistic competence could damage that confidence seriously. (the *Guardian*, 14 March 1989, p. 27)

Slowly but increasingly, the value of bilingualism (and multilingualism) is being recognized, not just for British ethnic minorities but also for the native speakers of first-language English who constitute the majority. As Edwards *et al.* (1988, p. 82) contend, the benefits to a society from having bilingual, biliterate people in it are increasingly acknowledged, though that acknowledgment is still accorded more readily with regard to European languages than to Asian and other minority languages. From the USA, Smith (1983) suggests that how English is being used in most of the world makes the title 'English as an International and International Language' (EIIL) more accurate than 'English to Speakers of Other Languages' (ESOL) embracing 'English as a Foreign Lan-guage' (EFL) and 'English as a Second Language' (ESL). He argues that 'English can and should be de-nationalized'. It could then become an inter-national auxiliary language (EIAL) for any country wishing to teach it. This is to some extent recognition of what is in fact happening. It adds to the international preference for English over other languages in competition for other-language status without necessarily affecting the status of foreign languages in Britain. Renate Bartsch hopes that the 'version of one of the many varieties of the super-variety International English' in which her *Norms of Language* is written – that is, 'the German variety of English' – will not 'discourage native English readers' (1987, Preface, ix).

According to a Scottish Education Department document (1946/88, p. 86), a much earlier Scottish official memorandum made a 'remarkable pronounce-ment' that 'The knowledge of a language other than the mother tongue is not a necessary part of the equipment of an educated mind.' Even if this meant specifically English and not *any* mother tongue (such as Lallans, Scots), it would be hard to take it seriously – except that the same bizarre opinion has recently been revived. Many people will not be surprised to find Sir Alfred Sherman, co-founder of the Centre for Policy Studies, expressing the narrow-minded view that 'Anyone born with English as his or her native language does not need other languages, in the sense that Greeks, Dutch, Danes and Spaniards do' (Sherman, 1989). But it *is* surprising that Sir Christopher Ball, chairman of the National Advisory Board for Public Higher Education – admittedly expressing a personal opinion (in *TES* 28 October 1988, p. 17) – offers breathtaking assertions in support of being monoglot – provided the 'mono' language is English! 'It is possible to be a civilized and educated person while speaking and understanding only English; it is increasingly difficult to be civilized and educated if one cannot speak and understand English.' His conclusion – that 'foreign languages have no place in the *compulsory core*-curriculum for speakers of English' (emphasis added) – merely endorses the official exclusion of modern languages from the tripartite core of subjects. His swingeing generalizations seem, with unnecessary excess, to deny the claims of modern foreign languages as foundation or additional subjects, where they are in fact listed. 'Making people learn unwillingly what they know they don't need' is admittedly – and almost by definition – 'bad education'. But to assert that 'Only a few of us need to be competent in foreign languages – for diplomacy, marketing, teaching, and similar specialized purposes' is tanta-mount to denying that to know and understand foreign cultures needs some knowledge of their languages and therefore of their ways of thought. Underlying Ball's simplistic case runs the isomorphic one-for-one fallacy discussed above.

It is probably not so much linguistic issues as an intuitive chauvinism ('vociferous and unthinking patriotism', in one dictionary's definition) that has caused our Prime Minister to condemn the original Lingua programme, promot-ing the learning of two foreign languages, as 'an infringement of national sovereignty' (*TES*, 28 May 1989, A2). Her Education Minister (Angela Rum-bold) has, however, ventured at least to modify the Thatcherite line for paradoxi-cally Thatcherite reasons. Speaking to delegates at the UK Centre for European Education conference, she asserted that 'to compete successfully in Europe' and 'to win our way in a competitive world', British complacency to foreign language learning must change. She commended (in the familiar official jargon) – as part of the 'European Dimension' – two 'initiatives', the European Awareness project in 12 UK local authorities and the European Studies Project extending educational co-operation between England, the two Irelands, Belgium, France and West Germany (*DES News* 336/89, 7 November 1989).

It is understandable that teachers of foreign languages, limited to four or five brief lessons each week, can find themselves – in Eric Hawkins's famous phrase – 'gardening in the gale of English' and can, as he writes, in his Introduction to a recent symposium of essays on intensive language teaching and learning, regard the first need to be of a 'wind-break' against the 'gale of English' (Hawkins 1988, p. 8). But too strong an exclusion of the native language could operate against language awareness, which should exploit the interpenetrations of languages, using all the linguistic resources available in the classroom. This is specially true for the many classes attended not only by single individual teachers of foreign European languages but also nowadays often by pupils (as well as teachers) speaking a wide range of 'ethnic minority' languages.

Some surprise has been expressed that 'there is no mention at all [in the Inspectorate's *English 5–16]* of the Language Awareness movement' (Stubbs, 1985, p. 26). The English Working Group's *English for ages 5 to 11* (DES and Welsh Office, 1988b) does not refer to any *movement* (either as a general tendency or as an organized *Movement*) but it frequently uses the term 'awareness' in its Report. In a paragraph on language acquisition (as relevant to linguistic terminology) it acknowledges acquisition as a 'common topic on many language awareness courses' (DES, 1988b, para. 5.37). A Reading Attainment Target is aimed at demonstrating 'awareness of language in the environment' (DES, 1988b, para. 9.12). Drama can extend 'awareness of language in use' (DES, 1988b, para. 14.7). The term 'awareness', not explicitly but by context collocated with 'language', occurs in:

para. 2.5   quoting (from Allen, 1988) teachers' need of 'a sensitive awareness of when to intervene and when to leave alone';

para. 3.11   school-leavers should have developed 'an awareness of some of the basic properties of human languages and their role in societies';

para. 5.7   children's 'metalinguistic awareness' (revealed in their uses of language in the extracts quoted) and the teacher's role in developing such awareness;

page 50   the Spelling Attainment Target II (no. 3) includes 'growing awareness of word families and their relationships'.

The importance of multilanguage awareness is recognized at some length in the Report's sections on 'English and other languages' (part of Chapter 3) and 'Bilingual Children' (Chapter 12).

To the emphasis on not teaching English 'in complete isolation' (p. 14 above) both Cox reports add insistence that *all* pupils, bilingual and monoglot, can benefit from multilingual experience:

> The evidence shows that such [bilingual] children will make greater progress in English if they know that their knowledge of their mother tongue is valued, if it is recognised that their experience of language is likely to be greater than that of their monoglot peers and, indeed, if their knowledge and experience can be put to good use in the classroom to the benefit of all pupils to provide examples of the structure and syntax of different languages, to provide a focus of discussion about language forms and for contrast and comparison with the structure of the English language (DES, 1988b, para. 12.9; DES, 1989, para. 10.12)

The NCLE Language Awareness Working Party has published a range of materials, variously contributed by teachers of English and of foreign languages. Problems of translation do not seem to figure largely in these materials and one would not expect them to do so with younger pupils. However, the older classes in primary schools, especially when they include speakers of non-English mother tongues, might multilingually explore common topics such as food, road signs, nursery rhymes and fairy tales. With secondary school students embarked upon modern language study, the versions of 'Jabberwocky' in English, French and German could lead on to quotations from other translations of *Alice*, of which there are nearly fifty. *Alice in many tongues*, edited by the American scholar Warren Weaver (1964), is illustrated with pictures and quotations of text from Swedish, Bengali, Thai, Croatian, Hebrew, Japanese and Danish translations.

Obviously, the languages brought into classrooms will vary according to the 'ethnic' constitution of classes as well as the ages of students. A sixth form that includes several speakers of Chinese could consider the status of word classes. For English, analysis has traditionally relied on the categories called (not altogether satisfactorily) parts of speech, but Chinese apparently manages without an equivalent apparatus. Ogden (1932, p. cx) of Basic English fame, reports that the Chinese have no verbs or parts of speech at all to correspond to things, processes, etc. He quotes from A. D. Sheffield an example to demonstrate this:

Ch'u men pu tai ch'ien
Pu ju chia li hsien

Go(ing) abroad without (tak)ing cash
(is) not up-to loaf(ing) at home.

Artificial languages

Ogden and Richards's Basic English, itself not a foreign language, is a simplified English language with a minimum of 850 words. Being man-made, it reminds one of artificial languages. Several hundred such are recorded, but most of them, devised in and since the nineteenth century, 'are based on elements drawn from natural languages' (Crystal, 1987b, p. 352). Esperanto, though not very widely used, is the best known of its kind. For teachers of English, it is probably easier than Interlingua, but that has also been used for serious work. A Swedish biochemist used it for writing about the threat of world famine. His prospectus (quoted in Bolinger, 1975, p. 595) reads:

Le Grande Fame: Un Stato de Guerra
Nos pote jam hodie facer observationes indicante que le etate del grande fame de facto ha comenciate. Nos pote p.ex. in certe paises 'developpante' observar le immigration del regiones rural al grande urbes, le quales se expande enormemente, p.ex. Bombay e Calcutta. Le resultato essera super-population, morte de fame, penuria, demonstrationes e revolutiones.

Adjuta per le paises industrial es necesse e ha jam comenciate in multe paises. Ma le situation es ben remarcabile, e mesmo cynic, pro que le paises povre sovente demanda armas in loco de cereales. Si le paises industrial seriosemente repartira viveres e material in mesura effective pro uso pacific, illos debera ipse reducer lor proprie standard de vita in grado considerabile.

Le adjuta debe obviente concentrar se a regiones que, recipiente contribution de materiales e viveres, pote possibilemente ipse meliorar lor situation, de modo que illos essera auto-sustenente.

Interlingua, like many other European artificial languages, depends heavily upon *cognate* words. It draws on lexical items that are identical or similar in form and meaning in the natural languages they come from. These languages are cognate in the sense that they make up a family of languages. The European Romance family has Latin as its linguistic 'father', with 'daughter' languages (such as Italian, French, Spanish) that are 'sisters' of each other. Cognate sequences – syntactic as well as semantic – are demonstrable in English sentences such as 'Examinations examine examinees', 'One hopes to do good deeds', and – less formally obvious – 'to run a successful race'. Bilingual dictionaries reveal the cognate vocabulary items shared by two languages. Some of these are deceptively cognate and therefore can lead to misunderstandings. The French-English ones are the *faux amis* discussed above (p. 37). We are told that these two languages have about eleven times more true than false cognates (Hammer, 1978, quoted by Ringbom, 1987, p. 59). The frequency of deceptive cognates hinders learning, whereas the existence of true cognates can facilitate it. We are naturally inclined, as Henry Sweet remarked (1964, p. 54), 'to assume that the nearer the foreign language is to our own, the easier it is'. But Ringbom (1987, p. 44) warns us that

> this very likeness is often a source of confusion. It is a help to the beginner who merely wants to understand the allied language, and is contented with a rough knowledge; but it is a hindrance to any thorough knowledge, because of the constant cross-associations that are sure to present themselves.

Language awareness would favour increased attention to such cross-associations. It would also attend to the frequency and nature of the borrowing of 'loan-words'. What Jespersen described as the 'linguistic omnivorousness' of English has developed enormously during the twentieth century. It is relevant for language teachers (and their students) to consider questions about the linguistic and cultural need for large-scale use of loan-words. The most obvious cases are of borrowing words to refer to 'things' and experiences missing (at least originally) from the receiving culture ('guillotine', 'falsetto', 'rucksack', 'eisteddfod', 'yashmak', 'samovar' and 'robot', to name but a few). These loans are so familiar that they are not normally italicized in print. Others – less used, more specialized and more foreign-looking – tend to retain the italics given to their first appearance in English (e.g., *leitmotiv, langlauf, entente, czardas, macramé*). There seems to be a positive correlation between 'culture-specificity' and untranslatableness. It is neither possible nor necessary to Anglicize the forms of 'sari' or 'muezzin' or 'mah-jong'.

The borrowing of words from foreign languages to fill gaps in the English language seems as reasonable as it is inevitable. But, as a glance at the English prose used by novelists and journalists reveals, our omnivorousness goes far beyond gap-filling. The so-called 'higher' journalism, given a serious topic, is often peppered with borrowings less easy to regard as necessary. In a few paragraphs of a review of a biography of Eric Gill, for instance, Bernard Levin (1989) 'borrows' *'outré'*, *'droit de seigneur'*, *'tout pardonner'*, *'paterfamilias'* and mentions Solon's law, thereby referring to *'nil de mortuis nisi bonum'*. One character in a short story by Georgina Hammick is a man for whom 'all invoices are, *per se* and *ipso facto* (if *a priori*) *pro forma*, all payments *ex gratia*, all evidence *prime facie*, all quids *pro quo* . . .'. He tells his wife to stop worrying, *nil desperandum*. Certainly most of these phrases are difficult to translate into equivalently crisp English forms. On the other hand, 'That goes without saying' is literally and satisfactorily equivalent to *'Ça va sans dire'*. To use the latter smacks somewhat of what Lewis Carroll commented on long ago as a tendency 'to regard utterances in foreign languages with deferential respect and reverential awe' (Sutherland, 1970, p. 222). Geoffrey Hughes (1988, p. 229) uses 'dissociation' to name 'the borrowing of opaque foreign terms [from soon after the Conquest] . . . often for motives of pretence and obfuscation'.

For teachers of English, the social-class implications of using 'unnecessary' foreign phrases to impress may be related to the conspicuous proliferation of foreign phrases in promotional advertising – for example, the well-known 'Vorsprung durch Technik'. When the Audi agency asked whether this 'ad' slogan would be added to the *Oxford English Dictionary*, John Simpson replied (1989, p. 60) that, though there was no lexicographical reason for excluding it, it would be omitted for not yet having passed into general currency. For teachers of foreign languages, the value of 'trawling' for foreign terms in modern English writing, and even in English dictionaries, should be more immediately useful.

Remorseless language change blurs distinctions between 'foreign' and 'non-foreign'. Foreign words can, in the modern jargon, 'go native'. In the latest version of Gowers's (1987, p. 75) *Complete Plain Words*, it is observed that 'Perhaps *sub judice, recherché, fait accompli* and *ad infinitum* are at the stage that *et cetera, agenda, garage* and *hotel* passed some time ago'. Bliss's *Dictionary of Foreign Words and Phrases in Current English* (1966) includes *garage* because that word was first used in English no earlier than 1902 and 'for several years thereafter was printed either in italics or written quotation marks. Its pronunciation is by no means fully anglicized yet, though it will surely become so.'

Bibliography

(Items marked * are recommended for reading.)

*Aitchison, Jean (1981) *Language Change: Progress or Decay*, Fontana.

—— (1987) *Words in the Mind: an Introduction to the Mental Lexicon*, Blackwell.

*Allen, David (1988) *English, whose English?* NAAE.

Allen, J. P. B. and Pit Corder, S. (1973) *Readings for Applied Linguistics*, Vol. 1, Oxford University Press.

Amidon, E. and Hough, F. (eds) (1987) *Interaction Analysis*, Addison-Wesley.

Arakelian, Paul G. (1975) 'Punctuation in a Late Middle English Manuscript', *Neuphilologische Mitteilungen*, LXXVI.

Austin, J. L. (1962) *How to do Things with Words*, Clarendon Press.

Bacon, Francis (1971) *The Physical and Metaphysical Works*, Book 1, Bell.

Baker, G. P. and Hacker, P. M. S. (1984) *Language, Sense and Nonsense*, Blackwell.

Bakhtin, Michael (1981) *The Dialogic Imagination; Four Essays*, ed. Michael Holquist, University of Texas Press.

Ball, Sir Christopher (1988) 'Misplaced accent on languages', *Times Educational Supplement*, 28 October 1988.

Bar-Hillel, Yehoshua (1956) 7th International Congress of Linguistics, King's College, London. Plenary session 11: Philosophy, Logic, and Social Anthropology, discussion.

*Barnes, D., Britton, J. N. and Rosen, H. (1969) *Language, the learner and the school*, Penguin.

*—— (1971) *Language, the learner and the school*, rev. edn, Penguin.

*Barnes, D., Britton, J. N. and Torbe, M. (1986) *Language, the learner and the school*, 3rd edn, Penguin.

Barney, Stephen A. (1977) *Word-hoard; an Introduction to Old English vocabulary*, Yale University Press.

Baron, Dennis E. (1982) *Grammar and Good Taste – reforming the English Language*, Yale University Press.

Bartsch, Renate (1987) *Norms of Language*, Longman.

de Beauvoir, Simone (1958) *Memoire d'une jeune fille rangée*, Gallimard.

Bellack, A. A. *et al.* (1966) *The Language of the Classroom*, Teachers College, Columbia University.

Berlin, B. and Kay, Paul (1969) *Basic Color Terms: their universality and evolution*, Berkeley, University of California.

Blamires, Harry (1950) *Repair the Ruins*, Bles.

Bloch, B. and Trager, G. L. (1942) *Outline of Linguistic Analysis*, Baltimore.

Bloomfield, Leonard (1933) *Language*, Holt.

Bolinger, Dwight (1968, 2nd edn 1975) *Aspects of Language*, Harcourt Brace Jovanovich.

Bosker, A. (1947) 'Some Aspects of the Study of Syntax', *Neophilologus*.

Bourne, Jill (1988) ' "Natural Acquisition" and a "Masked Pedagogy" ', *Applied Linguistics*, 9(1), March.

Boyd, William (1924) *Measuring Devices in Composition, Spelling and Arithmetic*, Harrap.

Britton, James N. (1977) 'Language and the Nature of Learning', in Squire (ed.) 1977.

—— *et al.* (1975) *The Development of Writing Abilities, 11–18*, Schools Council Research Studies, Macmillan.

Bronckart, J.-P. (1985) *The Language Sciences: an educational challenge?* UNESCO.

Brumfit, Christopher (1988) 'Responses to Kingman: a symposium', *English in Education*, 22(3), Autumn.

Brunelle, Eugene A. (1973) 'The biology of meaning', *Journal of Creative Behavior*, 7(1).

Bruner, Jerome (1975) 'Language as an Instrument of Thought', in Davies (ed.) (1975).

* Burchfield, Robert (1985) *The English Language*, Oxford University Press.

Butler, Christopher (1985) *Systemic Linguistics: Theory and Application*, Batsford.

Campbell, Jeremy (1982) *Grammatical Man*, Penguin.

Canham, G. W. (ed.) (1972) *Mother-Tongue Teaching*, UNESCO Institute for Education, Hamburg.

Carter, Ronald (ed.) (1982) *Linguistics and the Teacher*, RKP.

—— and McCarthy, Michael (1988) *Vocabulary and Language Teaching*, Longman.

Catford, J. C. (1959) 'English as a Foreign Language', in *The Teaching of English*, Communication Research Centre, Secker & Warburg.

—— (1965) *A Linguistic Theory of Translation*, Oxford University Press.

* Chace, Howard L. (1956) *Anguish Languish*, Prentice Hall.

Chafe, Wallace (1968) 'Review of Lamb's *Outline of Stratificational Grammar*', *Language*, 44(3), September, 593–603.

Chanan, Gabriel (ed.) (1973) *Towards a Science of Teaching*, NFER.

Chapman, Raymond (1988) 'We gonna rite wot we wonna', *English Today* 14, IV(2), 39–42.

Cherry, Colin (1957) *On Human Communication*, MIT Press.

Chiu, Rosaline K. (1973) 'Measuring Register Characteristics', *IRAL*, XI(1), 51–68.

Chomsky, Noam (1959) 'A Review of B. F. Skinner's *Verbal Behavior*' in *Language*, 35(1), 26–58.

—— (1966) *Cartesian Linguistics*, Harper & Row.

—— (1968) *Language and Mind*, Harcourt Brace.

Clark, H. H. and Clark, E. V. (1977) *Psychology and Language: an Introduction to Psycholinguistics*, Harcourt Brace.

Clout, Celia (1987) 'The Best and Worst of Times', *Use of English*, 39(1).

Coleridge, S. T. (1884) *The Table Talk and Omnia* (ed. Ashe), Bell.

Committee for Linguistics in Education (1984) *Guidelines for Evaluating School Instruction about Language*, CLIE.

Coulthard, Malcolm (1977) *An Introduction to Discourse Analysis*, Longman.

Crick, Bernard (1981) *George Orwell: A Life*, Secker & Warburg.

Cruse, D. A. (1986) *Lexical Semantics*, Oxford University Press.

Crystal, David (1969) *Journal of Linguistics*, 6(2), 302.

* Crystal, David (1980) *A First Dictionary of Linguistics and Phonetics*, Deutsch.

—— (1984) *Who Cares About English Usage?*, Penguin.

—— (1987a) *Child Language, Learning and Linguistics*, 2nd edn, Edward Arnold.

—— (1987b) *Cambridge Encyclopedia of Language*, Cambridge University Press.

—— and Davy, D. (1973) *Investigating English Style*, Longman.

Czerniewska, Pam (1988) 'Objectives for Language Learning', in Jones and West, pp. 123–32.

Davies, Alan (ed.) (1975) *Problems of Language and Learning*, Heinemann.

—— (1977) *Language & Learning in Early Childhood*, Heinemann.

—— and Widdowson, H. G. (1974) 'Reading and writing', in Allen, J. P. G. and Corder, S. Pit, *Techniques in Applied Linguistics* (Edinburgh Course in Applied Linguistics, Vol. 3).

Derrida, Jacques (1976) *Grammatology* (trans. Spivak), Johns Hopkins University Press.

*DES (Department of Education and Science) (1975) *A Language for life* (the Bullock Report), HMSO.

*—— (1979) *Aspects of Secondary Education in England: a survey by H. M. Inspectors of Schools*, HMSO.

*—— (1984) *English from 5 to 16, Curriculum Matters 1*, HMSO.

*—— (1985a) *The Curriculum from 5 to 16*, HMSO.

*—— (1985b) *Education for All* (Swann Report: Inquiry into the Education of Children from Ethnic Minority Groups), HMSO.

*—— (1986) *English from 5 to 16: the Responses to Curriculum Matters 1, an HMI Report*, HMSO.

*—— (1988) *Report of the Committee of Inquiry into the Teaching of the English Language* (Kingman Report), HMSO.

*—— and Welsh Office (1987) *The National Curriculum*, July.

—— (1988a) *National Curriculum: Task Group in Assessment and Testing* (Black Report), HMSO.

*—— (1988b) *National Curriculum: English for ages 5 to 11* (Cox Report 1), November, HMSO.

*—— (1989) *National Curriculum: English for ages 5 to 16* (Cox Report 2), June, HMSO.

Diack, Hunter (1955) *Nottingham Institute Bulletin No. 20*, May.

Dinneen, Francis (1967) *An Introduction to General Linguistics*, Holt, Rinehart, and Winston.

*Doughty, P., Pearce, J. and Thornton, G. (1971) *Language in Use*, Edward Arnold.

Eco, Umberto (1976) *A Theory of Semiotics*, Indiana University Press.

Edwards, A. D. and Westgate, D. P. G. (1987) *Investigating Classroom Talk*, Falmer Press.

Edwards, Carole *et al.* (1988) 'Language or English? The needs of bilingual pupils', in Jones and West.

Eisner, O. and Tucker, S. (1965) *Language and Education* (Lyndale House Papers), Bristol University Institute of Education.

Fishman, Joshua A. (1973) 'The Sociology of Language', in Miller, G. A. (ed.).

Flanders, Ned (1963) 'Intent, Action and Feedback: a preparation for teaching', *Journal of Teacher Education*, 14, 251–60.

—— (1970) *Analyzing Teaching Behavior*, Addison-Wesley.

Flowerden, John (1988) 'Speech acts and language teaching', *Language Teaching*, 21(2) April, 69–82

*Fowler, H. W. and F. G. (1906) *The King's English*, Oxford University Press.
Francis, Nelson (1973) 'Revolution in Grammar', in Savage, J. K., *Linguistics for Teachers*, Science Research Associates, Chicago.
Fromkin, Victoria and Rodman, R. (1978) *An Introduction to Language*, International/2nd edn, Holt, Rinehart & Winston.
*Gardner, Martin (ed.) (1965, rev. 1970) *The Annotated Alice*, Penguin.
Gatherer, W. A. (1980) *A Study of English*, Heinemann.
Goldberg, I. (1938) *The Wonder of Words*, Appleton-Century.
Goodman, K. and Goodman, Y. (1988) 'Learning about Psycholinguistic Processes by Analyzing Oral Reading', in Mercer (ed.), Vol. 2, pp. 163–71.
*Gowers, Sir Ernest (1987) *The Complete Plain Words*, 3rd edn, revised by S. Greenbaum and J. Whitcut. Penguin.
Graustein, G. *et al.* (1977) *English Grammar*, Leipzig.
Gregory, M. and Carroll, S. (1978) *Language and Situation: language varieties in their social contexts*, RKP.
Grice, H. P. (1957) 'Meaning', *Philosophical Review*, 66.
——(1981) 'Presupposition and conventional implicatures', in Cole, P. (ed.), *Radical Pragmatics*, Academic Press.
Grierson, Herbert J. G. (1944) *Rhetoric and English Composition*, Oliver & Boyd.
Griffith, Peter (1987) *Literary Theory and English Teaching*, Open University Press.
Halliday, M. A. K. (1978) *Language as Social Semiotic*, Edward Arnold.
——(1985) *An Introduction to Functional Grammar*, Edward Arnold.
——McIntosh, A. and Strevens, P. (1964) *The Linguistic Sciences and Language Teaching*, Longman.
Hammer, P. (1978) 'The Utility of Cognates in Second Language Acquisition', Paper read at 5th AILA Congress, Montreal.
Harding, Rosamond (1967) *An Anatomy of Inspiration*, Barnes & Noble.
Harris, Roy (1986) *The Origin of Writing*, Duckworth.
——(1987) *The Language Machine*, Duckworth.
——(1989) 'Who Will Translate the Translators', *Encounter*, February.
*Hawkins, Eric (1984) *Awareness of Language: an Introduction*, Cambridge University Press, 1984, rev. 1987.
——(ed.) (1988) *Intensive Language Teaching and Learning*, CILT.
Hockett, C. F. (1967) *Language, Mathematics, and Linguistics*, Mouton.
——(1968) *The State of the Art*, Mouton.
——(1977) 'The Problem of Universals', in *The View from Language: selected essays 1948–1974*, University of Georgia Press.
Hopkins, Mary Francis (1989) 'The Rhetoric of Heteroglossia in Flannery O'Connor's "Wise Blood"', *Quarterly Journal of Speech*, 75, 198–211.
Hudson, Richard (1982) 'Some Issues over which Linguists can Agree', in Carter (ed.), 1982.
*Hughes, Geoffrey (1988) *Words in Time: A Social History of the English Vocabulary*, Blackett.
Huizinga, J. (1935) *In the Shadow of Tomorrow*, Heinemann.
Incorporated Association of Assistant Masters (1952) *The Teaching of English*, Cambridge University Press.
Jakobson, Roman (1960) 'Closing statement: linguistics and poetics', in Sebeok, T. A. (ed.) *Style in Language*, MIT Press, p. 139.

James, C. V. (1979) 'Foreign Languages in the School Curriculum', *Foreign Languages in Education*, CILT.

Jeffreys, M. V. C. (1955) *Beyond Neutrality*, Pitman.

Jones, M. and West, A. (1988) *Learning Me Your Language*, Mary Glasgow Publications, 1988.

Joos, Martin (1962) *The Five Clocks*, Harcourt Brace.

Kirkup, James (1959) *Memoirs of a Dutiful Daughter*, translation of de Beauvoir's *Memoires d'une jeune fille rangée*, Deutsch and Weidenfeld and Nicolson (Penguin, 1963).

Knight, Roger (1989) 'A Utopian English', the *Guardian*, 25 July.

Koessler, Maxime and Derocquigny, Jules (1928) *Les Faux-amis ou les trahisons du vocabulaire anglais*, Vuibert.

Kreidler, Charles W. (1989) *The Pronunciation of English*, Blackwell.

Labov, W. (1972) 'Where do Grammars Stop?' in Shuy, R. W. (ed.), *Sociolinguistics: current trends and prospects*, 23rd Annual Round Table Meeting, Georgetown.

Lakoff, George (1975) 'Hedges: a study in meaning criteria and the logic of fuzzy concepts', in Hockney, D. J., Harper, W. and Freed, B., *Contemporary Research in Philosophical Logic and Linguistic Semantics*, D. Reidel.

—— and Johnson, Mark (1980) *Metaphors We Live By*, University of Chicago Press.

Land, Stephen R. (1986) *The Philosophy of Language in Britain*, Ams Press.

de Landscheere, G. (1973) 'Analysis of Verbal Interaction in the Classroom', in Chanan (ed.) 1973, pp. 60–84.

Langer, Suzanne (1962) *Philosophical Sketches*, Mentor.

Lawlor, Sheila (1988) *Correct Core: simple curricula for English, mathematics and science*, Centre for Policy Studies, No. 93.

—— (1989) 'Funding the Arts', *Encounter*, January.

Leech, Geoffrey (1969) *Towards a Semantic Description of English*, Longmans.

—— (1974) *Semantics*, Penguin.

—— (1983) *Principles of Pragmatics*, Longmans.

Leeds, Chris (1988) 'Parlez-vous Business?', *Modern Languages*, 69(3), September, 179–86.

Levin, Bernard (1989) 'Taking Gill's True Measure', *The Times*, 13 March, p. 16.

Lewis, C. S. (1967) *Studies in Words*, Cambridge University Press.

Lloyd, D. Y. and Warfel, H. R. (1956) *American English in its Cultural Setting*, Knopf.

Lott, Bernard (1988) 'Language and Literature', *Language Teaching*, 21(1), January.

Lounsbury, Thomas R. (1908) *The Standard of Usage in English*, Harper.

Lyons, John (1981a) *Language, Meaning and Context*, Fontana.

—— (1981b) 'Structural Semantics in Retrospect', in Hope, T. E. *et al.* (eds), *Language, Meaning and Style*, Leeds University Press.

Marland, Michael (1980) Foreword to Robertson (1980).

don marquis (1934) *archy's life of mehitabel*, Faber.

Martinet, A. (1960) *Elements of General Linguistics*, Faber.

Mayper, Stewart A. (1986–7) 'Who Only English Know', *General Semantics Bulletin*.

Meek, Margaret and Miller, Jane (eds) (1984) *Changing English: essays for Harold Rosen*, Heinemann Educational for University of London Institute of Education.

Mencken, H. L. (1936) *The American Language*, 4th edn, Knopf (first published 1919).

*Mercer, Neil (ed.) (1988) *Language and Literacy from an Educational Perspective*, 2 vols, Open University Press.

Meredith, G. P. (1956) 'Semantics in Relation to Psychology', *Archivum Linguisticum*, Vol. 8, Fascicule 1.

Messer, Bill (1976) 'A Lesson for the Teacher', in Torbe, Michael and Protherough, Robert: *Classroom Encounters*, Ward Lock Educational.

Michael, Ian (1987) *The Teaching of English: From the sixteenth century to 1870*, Cambridge University Press.

Miller, G. A. (ed.) (1973) *Communication, Language, and Meaning*, Basic Books.

—— and Johnson-Laird, P. (1976) *Language and Perception*, Cambridge University Press.

Mitchell, Rosamond (1988) *Communicative Language Teaching in Practice*, CILT.

Mittins, W. H. (1962) 'Marking Composition', in Jackson, B. and Thompson, D. (eds), *English in Education*, Chatto & Windus.

—— (1988) *The Naming of Parts*, NATE.

—— Salu, Mary, Edminson, Mary, and Coyne, Sheila (1970) *Attitudes to English Usage*, Oxford University Press.

Mobley, Maureen (1987) *Working Paper No. 5*, Secondary Examinations Council, p. 5.

Moffett, James (1968) *Teaching the Universe of Discourse*, Houghton Mifflin.

Mooij, J. J. A. (1976) *A Study of Metaphor*, North-Holland.

Morris, Charles (1946) *Signs, Language, and Behavior*, Prentice Hall.

Nash, Walter (1986) *English Usage*, Routledge & Kegan Paul.

Nuttall, Desmond (1969) 'Test "monster" must be killed says professor', *Times Educational Supplement*, 10 March 1989, A1.

O'Donnell, W. R. and Todd, Loreto (1980) *Variety in Contemporary English*, Allen & Unwin.

Ogden, C. K. (1932) *Bentham's Theory of Fictions*, Routledge & Kegan Paul.

—— and Richards, I. A. (1923) *The Meaning of Meaning*, Routledge & Kegan Paul.

Ortony, Andrew (ed.) (1979) *Metaphor and Thought*, Cambridge University Press.

Osgood, C. E., Suci, G. J. and Tannenbaum, P. H. (1957) *The Measurement of Meaning*, University of Illinois.

Passmore, John (1970) *Perfectibility of Man*, Duckworth.

Pearce, John (1972) *School Examinations*, Collier-Macmillan.

Peddiwell, J. (1939) *Saber-toothed Curriculum*, McGraw-Hill.

Perera, Katharine (1987) *Understanding Language*, National Association of Advisers in English.

Peters, Margaret (1967) *Spelling: Caught or Taught?*, Routledge & Kegan Paul.

Popper, Karl (1976) *Unended Quest*, Fontana.

Potter, Stephen (ed.) (1954) *Sense of Humour*, Reinhardt.

Powell, Neil (1976) 'The End of English', *Use of English*, 28(1), 17–22.

Quirk, Randolph (1960) 'Towards a Description of English Usage', *Transactions of Philological Society*.

—— (1969) 'On Conceptions of Good Grammar', *Essays by Divers Hands*, NS, Vol. 35.

—— (1989) 'Separated by a common dilemma', *Times Higher Education Supplement*, 10 February, pp. 15–18.

Randall, John R. (1976) *The Making of the Modern Mind*, Columbia University Press.

Renfrew, Colin (1987) *Archaeology and Language*, Cape.

Richards, Ivor A. (1938) *Interpretation in Teaching*, Routledge & Kegan Paul.

Richmond, W. Kenneth (1967) *The Teaching Revolution*, Methuen.

Ringbom, Håkan (1987) *The Role of the First Language in Foreign Language Learning*, Multilingual Matters.

Robertson, Irene (1980) *Language across the Curriculum; four case studies* (Schools Council Working Paper 67), Methuen Educational.

Robins, R. H. (1951) *Ancient and Mediaeval Grammatical Theory in Europe*, Kinnikat Press.

—— (1964) *General Linguistics*, Longmans.

Rosten, Leo (1937, 1970) The Education of Hyman Kaplan, Penguin (1990).

—— (1959, 1968) The Return of Hyman Kaplan, Penguin (1968).

Ruby, L. (1956) *The Art of Making Sense*, Peter Davies.

Russell, Bertrand (1948) *Human Knowledge: its scope and limits*, Allen & Unwin.

Rutherford, William (1987) *Second Language Grammar Learning and Teaching*, Longman.

—— and Smith, S. (1988) *Grammar and Second Language Learning*, Newbury House.

Sadock, Jerrold M. (1979) 'Figurative Speech and Linguistics', in Ortony (ed.) (1979).

Salkie, Jerrold (1989) 'Linguistic Virtuosity', *Times Higher Education Supplement*, 31 March.

Salter, Michael (1987) 'Language – the Challenge of Change', *Modern Languages*, 68(2), June.

Sapir, Edward (1921) *Language*, Harcourt Brace.

—— (1924) *The Grammarian and His Language* in *Selected Writings of E. Sapir in Language, Culture, and Personality*, University of California Press, 1941.

Saporta, Sol (ed.) (1961) *Psycholinguistics – A Book of Readings*, Holt, Rinehart & Winston.

Saunders, George (1983) *Bilingual Children: guidance for the family*, Multilingual Matters.

Scottish Education Department (1946–58) *Secondary Education*, HMSO.

Sherman, Sir Alfred (1989) 'Language Matters', Newsletter of the Associated Examinations Board, reprinted in *Times Educational Supplement*, 13 October.

Simon, A. and Boyer, E. G. (1967) *Mirrors for Behaviour: an anthology of classroom observations*, Research for Better Schools, Philadelphia.

Simon, John (1981) *Paradigms Lost*, Chatto & Windus.

Simpson, John (1989) 'Words from the Front', *English Today* 18, 5(2), April.

Sinclair, John (1985) *Language Awareness in Six Easy Lessons*, National Congress on Languages in Education.

——, Forsyth, I. J., Coulthard, R. M. and Ashby, M. (1972) *The English Used by Teachers and Pupils* (SSRC Report), University of Birmingham.

Skelton, John (1988) 'The Care and Maintenance of Hedges', *English Language Teaching*, 42(1), January.

Skinner, B. F. (1957) *Verbal Behavior*, Appleton-Century-Crofts.

Sklar, Elizabeth S. (1976–7) 'The Possessive Apostrophe: the development and decline of a crooked mark', *College English*, Vol. 38.

Smith, Frank (1928/75) *Comprehension and Learning*, Holt, Rinehart & Winston.

Smith, Larry E. (ed.) (1983) *Readings in English as an International Language*, Pergamon.

Squire, J. R. (ed.) 1977) *The Teaching of English* (76th Yearbook of the National Society for the Study of English), University of Chicago Press.

Stein, Gertrude (1931/75) *How to Write*, Dover Publications.

—— (1977) *How Writing is Written*, Black Sparrow Press.

Steiner, George (1975) *After Babel*, Oxford University Press.

Strang, Barbara M. H. (1970) *A History of English*, Methuen.

Strevens, Peter (1977) *New Orientations in the Teaching of English*, Oxford University Press.

—— (1985) 'Standards and the Standard Language', *English Today*, 2, April.

—— (1986) NCLE Language Awareness Working Paper, Newsletter No. 6, June.

—— (ed.) (1965) *Five Inaugural Lectures*, Oxford University Press.

Stubbs, Michael (1976) *Language, Schools and Classrooms*, Methuen.

—— (1980) *Language and Literacy: the sociolinguistics*, Routledge & Kegan Paul.

—— (1985) British Association of Applied Linguistics, Newsletter No. 24, Autumn.

Sutherland, Robert D. (1970) *Language and Lewis Carroll*, Mouton.

Sweet, Henry (1899, 1964) *The Practical Study of Languages*, Oxford University Press.

ten Brinke, Steven (1986) *The complete mother tongue curriculum*, Longman.

Thody, Philip and Evans, Howard (1985) *Faux Amis and Key Words: a dictionary guide to French language, culture and society through lookalikes and confusables*, Athlone Press.

Torbe, Michael and Protherough, Robert (1976) *Classroom Encounters*, Ward Lock Educational.

Trim, J. L. M. (1975) 'Weighing up your Words', *Times Higher Education Supplement*, 28 March.

Tsur, Reuven (1975) 'Two Critical Attitudes', *College English*, 36 (7) March.

Tucker, Susie (1972) *Enthusiasm: A Study in Semantic Change*, Cambridge University Press.

Veblen, Thorsten (1899) *The Theory of the Leisure Class*, first British edition Allen & Unwin, 1925.

Vigotsky, L. S. (1961) 'Thought and Speech', in Saporta (ed.), 1961.

Walpole, Hugh (1941) *Semantics – The Nature of Words and their Meanings*, W. W. Norton.

Wardhaugh, Ronald (1986) *An Introduction to Sociolinguistics*, Blackwell.

Warren, A. and Wellek, K. (1949) *Theory of Literature*, Cape.

*Watson, Ken (1981, rev. 1987) *English Teaching in Perspective*, Open University Press.

Weaver, Warren (1964) *Alice in many Tongues*, University of Wisconsin Press.

Welby, Victoria (1903) *What is Meaning? Studies in the Development of Significance*, Macmillan.

Wells, Gordon (1974) *Language Development in Pre-School Children*, University of Bristol School of Education.

*Welsh Office (1989) *Welsh for ages 5 to 16*, HMSO.

White, R. V. (1974) 'Communicative Competence – Registers and Second Language Teaching', *IRAL*, XII(2), May.

Whitehead, A. N. (1932) *Aims of Education*, Williams & Northgate.

—— (1933) *Adventures of Ideas*, Cambridge University Press.

—— (1948) *Essays in Science and Philosophy*, Rider.

Whorf, Benjamin Lee (1956) *Language, Thought, and Reality*, MIT Press.

Widdowson, H. G. (1979) *Explorations in Applied Linguistics*, Oxford University Press.

—— (1983) 'New Starts and Different Kinds of Failure', in Freedman, A., Pringle, I. and Yalden, J., *Learning to Write: first language / second language*, Longman.

Wilkins, David A. (1972) *Linguistics in Language Teaching*, Edward Arnold.

Wilkinson, A. M. (1971) *The Foundations of Language*, Oxford University Press.

Wragg, E. C. (1973) 'A Study of Student Teachers in the Classroom', in Chanan (ed.).

Index